SO-BNA-723

DOUBLE VISION

Alexandra Dundas Todd

DOUBLE VISION

AN EAST-WEST COLLABORATION FOR COPING WITH CANCER

SETON HALL UNIVERSITY
WALSH LIBRARY
SO. ORANGE, N.J.

Wesleyan University Press
Published by University Press of New England
Hanover and London

RC
280
·B7
T63
1994

Wesleyan University Press
Published by University Press of New England
Hanover, NH 03755
© 1994 by Alexandra Todd and John Andrew Todd, Jr.
All rights reserved
Printed in the United States of America   5   4   3   2   1
CIP data appear at the end of the book

Excerpts from the book in an earlier form appeared in the
March 1993 issue of *Sojourner: The Women's Forum.*

For All the Practitioners,
Eastern and Western, Who Helped

"And twofold Always. May God us keep
From Single vision & Newton's sleep!"

WILLIAM BLAKE, 1802

CONTENTS

Contents

ACKNOWLEDGMENTS

When friends heard about the research I did to help my son, Drew, cope with cancer, they encouraged me to write about it. As a medical sociologist and writer, they argued, I could provide valuable information to others—both people who are ill and those who want to stay healthy. My response was a certain "no." How could either I or Drew relive such a troubling time? That said, one night while sitting at the kitchen table I started writing. I couldn't stop. I became caught up in what some survivors of trauma call an "autobiographical imperative." Perhaps I was "hoping to purge the horrors" as Afrikaner poet Breyten Breytenback, once jailed for his antiapartheid activities, puts it.

By the time I finished writing the book, however, I was clear on its purposes. For myself, Drew, and our family, while I haven't purged the memories, I have given them "shape." For my friends and the reading public, I have gathered all my findings together in the hope that what helped Drew might help others. For researchers in medical sociology and health care, I hope to encourage more study into alternative medicines.

Acknowledgments

The following family members, friends, and colleagues offered suggestions and comments that helped make this book possible. Drew Todd read each draft, comparing his experience of events with mine, adding subtleties I couldn't have perceived without him. Stephen Fox edited the manuscript and helped me with everything else. To the other contributors I offer many thanks: Rebecca Green, Nicole Rafter, Jane Leserman, Catherine Ryan, Andy Todd, Sally Schwartz, Sarah Rose Todd, Bill Fishman, Eric Lichtman, Wendy Sanford, Sue Fisher, Nancy Waring, Pat Rieker, Elizabeth Driehaus, Vincent Cioffari, Valerie Blake, and Will Wright.

I am grateful to my colleagues at Suffolk University for their support of this project. Janice Fama spent extensive time on the manuscript at the computer; reference librarians Kathi Maio, Jim Coleman, Joe Middleton, and Kristin Djorup provided invaluable help with computer searches and tracking down obscure articles; and Michael Ronayne, Dean of the College of Liberal Arts and Sciences, generously gave me leave to care for Drew during his illness and a sabbatical afterward to write about it.

Finally, thanks to my agent, Robin Straus, for her work in promoting the manuscript, and Terry Cochran and Suzanna Tamminen, editors at Wesleyan University Press, for embracing the book with such enthusiasm and energy.

INTRODUCTION

The Chinese word for crisis consists of two characters: danger and opportunity. When my son, Drew, a senior in college, was diagnosed with a rare form of cancer bordering his brain, the danger was clear; the opportunity was less apparent. Danger flashed through our lives daily, while opportunities lay waiting in murky waters, to emerge only tentatively. Family closeness, the ability to savor each moment, to find strength and courage where we didn't know they existed, to discover new methods of treatment that complemented the surgeries and radiation and eased both body and mind, all contributed to making the unbearable bearable, turning an assault into a challenge.

Drew's story is a grim one with a happy ending. It is a story about cancer and recovery, about exploring the connections among heroic Western medical cures and gentle Eastern medical healings, about appreciating the bonds between mother and son, about the challenge of facing death and the joy of living. Drew's courage—not the stoicism of a John Wayne but the ability to shoulder shocks, look the unexpected in the eye with an expectant gaze, cope with the uncopable with a sense of irony as well as pathos—is a casual courage that is the heart of this book.

In a strange way this book is not about life versus death. It is more about the process of living, regardless of how long or brief life might be. It is about the moment and how precious each one is. It is about the struggle to remain an active participant in one's own life when out-of-control events make yielding a seductive force. It is about seeking the unknown, such as Eastern healing techniques, to combine with the more familiar surgery and radiation. It is about having the courage to grasp those unknowns and make them work for you.

As a medical sociologist I have studied and written about Western medicine, mostly about its problems, for fifteen years. My research has focused on the doctor-patient relationship and the workings of the Western medical model. More recently, I have incorporated alternative medical approaches into teaching, research, and my own health care (which I discuss in chapter 2). When Drew became ill, I had an arsenal of information to draw on. My hope in telling Drew's story—a story of personal experiences (early chapters), mingled with sociological research and analysis, of the usefulness, indeed the need, for combining the best of conventional medical techniques with the benefits of alternative, mostly Asian methods (later chapters)—is that it will help others, both those who are ill and want to feel better and those who are well and want to stay healthy.

For example, the Japanese, all too familiar with radiation after Hiroshima and Nagasaki, have done intriguing research on foods that work to eliminate excess radiation and toxins from the body. I believe these methods helped Drew bounce through eight weeks of intensive radiation, whereas others in his program suffered a host of ill effects. This information, invaluable to Drew, should be available to everyone. No prescription exists for wellness or for coping with illness. Each person's journey is a unique one. Drew's experiences simply add to the chronicles already told of ways that can help.

In one sense this book is Drew's story told in my voice, a story cancer survivors will recognize. It is also my story, the agony of a mother of a sick child (regardless of age), when for once you can't make it better, make everything all right—a story all parents will recognize if only in their fears.

Today, in the wake of Drew's crisis, the world does seem a more dangerous place, where anything can happen, a place where bad things do indeed happen to good people. But learning to live with that danger has sharpened our awareness, honed our senses to the opportunities to be grasped now in case the moment passes and the gold ring is forever missed.

DOUBLE VISION

Chapter One

CASUAL COURAGE

My friend Cathy says Drew has casual courage. Drew is my son, twenty-one years old, a senior in college. Since he was small, he's ventured into the world, confident it would welcome him, and it usually has. When he was four, for example, I took him to a friend's family barbecue. My friend warned me about her three large, unruly brothers-in-law. "If they were coming down the street, you would cross it," she told me. "Just ignore them. They'll be off drinking anyway." As we arrived, I noticed three enormous "most wanted" look-alikes loitering in the backyard drinking whiskey from a bottle, boasting scars and leather jackets. Drew saw them and headed straight for trouble. From the porch I saw his blond head look up at the men with an open grin and heard him ask, "What's happening, guys?" Not much as it turned out, as these toughs softened, put away their bottle, and played catch with him until dinner.

As he grew to adulthood, Drew's guileless ability to engage varieties of people in diverse situations continued to impress and often amaze me. He seemed to have little sense of danger, and thus when he became ill, it took him—took all of us—by surprise. He had been healthy all of his life. Nothing prepared us for the diagnosis, in September 1991, of a fast-growing, aggressive, large tumor in the sphenoid sinus area of his head, bordering his brain and settling on his optic nerve. We didn't even know he had a sphenoid sinus, the first of many new terms we could have lived happily knowing nothing about.

A year earlier, in the fall of 1990, Drew had gone to Washington, D.C., to intern in Congress for a semester. He started having sinus pain, diagnosed as an infection. One of his advisors reassured him: Washington is humid, built on swampland; newcomers often experience allergies, sinus troubles. But the pain continued, accompanied by fatigue and headaches. X rays showed no infection.

Drew, a government major, had planned carefully and waited a long time for this internship. As a high school student he had applied to be a page in Congress but had not been chosen. He had all of the routine qualifications. With a friend he had also started a political newspaper focused on issues such as AIDS and the draft, rather than writing for the official student paper, which spotlighted dances and new cars. He thought he had a shot at the job. He did. He was a runner-up. Now, a junior in college, he had his chance to work in government.

When Drew called to say he was missing classes and skipping out on Congressional meetings—all he wanted to do was sleep—I was surprised. It was unlike Drew to miss out on anything. He was always active, always an enthusiast, his optimism a contrast to my pessimism, his outgoing ways a foil to my diffidence. Drew sleeping all day? Drew withdrawing from political mayhem? Strange. But how serious can sinus pain be? In response to what now seem clear markers, I came up with the first of many misdiagnoses. As a medical sociologist, with fifteen years of thinking about health and illness, I thought I knew a lot—always a mistake.

I conferred with Drew's grandfather, a retired Washington doctor. I suggested mononucleosis. Blood work showed no mononucleosis and nothing else wrong for that matter. The headaches got worse. I suggested a recurrence of his childhood allergy to dairy foods. Doctors, reluctant to connect diet and nutrition to health, didn't pay much attention. A CAT scan was done (a scanning technique that combines computer and X-ray technologies). Nothing.

My husband, Stephen, Drew's stepfather, went to Washington on a research trip. While there he loaded Drew up with vitamins and discussed further the dairy-allergy possibility. Drew took the vitamins and stopped eating cheese, milk, and butter. He felt better; not great, but better. If he did nothing but required work and slept, he could manage. Gone was his enthusiasm to explore American government to the fullest; gone too was his social exuberance, his interest in making friends, in getting to know a new city and the college scene. His friend Rebecca went down to see him on occasional weekends. He mostly slept. Drew's father remembered that he had been unusually congested and pale all of the summer before, a summer spent in Santa Cruz, California, a town on the beach. But his energy and health had been fine. Dairy allergy, I proclaimed for the hundredth time. After all, the tests had been done; we could rule out anything serious.

Anyway, he was getting better. I was busy with health troubles of my own in Boston and decided to wait until Christmas vacation to pursue this further. But another symptom occurred—exceptionally dry skin. Dry skin in that humid city built on a swamp? Drew came home early for Thanksgiving. By that time his skin was driving him crazy with constant itching and breaking out in rashes from scratching. I sent him to our family doctor, who fit him into a busy preholiday schedule. Dry winter weather, he said. Common, he said. Use more lotion. Drew, frustrated by his increasingly untrustworthy body, bathed himself with lotions and took off to spend the rest of Thanksgiving vacation in northern New England with Rebecca and her family. There his skin went wild. Rebecca's father, a doctor at a university research center, called a dermatologist. This doctor said extreme dry skin and eczema had led to impetigo. He prescribed antibiotics for the impetigo and special soaps and lotion for the eczema. But he was puzzled. Such dry skin in someone with no history of this problem? Raging impetigo in someone Drew's age? Something didn't fit. These conditions, however, improved quickly with the medication. If the special products were used correctly, the scaling was kept at bay. That's all Drew wanted. He was getting tired of hearing "puzzled."

Health problems took a back seat to end-of-semester frenzy, both for Drew as a student and for me, a professor. Drew was especially excited about a paper he was writing on blues artist John Lee Hooker, and when I talked with him, that was his focus. His health receded further to the back of my mind.

At home for Christmas vacation, he seemed too thin, too pale, too tentative, but he was in good spirits. His head still hurt on and off, but he didn't mention it. He was basically sick of being sick.

On the morning before Christmas we were due to leave for a holi-

day with in-laws in New Hampshire. Drew woke up with the "flu"—
aches, fever, exhaustion, splitting headache. The flu *was* going around.
Oh well, we all laughed, this is not your year; 1991 has got to be better.

After Christmas, Drew and Rebecca went to California to see
Drew's father's family and ski. He left feeling fine. After the ski trip he
was going to Stanford Medical Center for a complete checkup. The
physician in Washington had already sent the CAT scan and various
medical records. By now Drew was so used to a low-grade headache, and
thankful when it wasn't severe, that background pain was normal.

Another round of workups produced a new and more satisfying, if
disquieting, diagnosis—cluster headaches. My trips to the library re-
vealed this to be a vague label but a common problem. The Stanford
neurologist prescribed a drug that helped. If he felt a headache coming
on and took the medication, he avoided the pain. We were relieved—the
unknown had turned into the known, even the controllable. Drew was
disconcerted that he had a chronic health problem but reassured that his
headaches could be stopped. I stubbornly held onto a possible dairy
allergy as a contributing factor in his health. His headaches did get worse
when he ate cheese, requiring more drugs. I also optimistically hoped
that this was something he would outgrow. In any case, we all relaxed.
We stopped our vigilance.

The new semester began. Drew was back at Connecticut College,
excited about his courses, glad to be out of a city he will always associate
with swampy sultriness. Life went on.

What I didn't know was that I should have been concerned. I didn't
know that all spring Drew spent little to no time with his friends. They
felt abandoned by him and thought Rebecca had become his only interest. In fact, Rebecca was his lifeline. I didn't know that she shook him
out of sleep to get him to class, regardless of how late his first class was;
that on nights when he didn't have the energy to get to the nearby
cafeteria, Rebecca brought him dinner; that he spent weekends watching
TV or sleeping rather than socializing. He became nearly a hermit, with
only one close friend, Rebecca, on a small, intimate college campus. This
especially confused his friends, to whom he had been such an outgoing,
involved companion, campaigning successfully for student office and
participating in varied intellectual, cultural, and social activities.

In fact I'd sometimes thought Drew was *too* social. The summer
after his freshman year, when he still felt fine, he rented a cottage on
Cape Cod with a group of friends—a tiny cottage with a lot of friends.

He and his friend "Bad Bill," as Stephen and I called him, got summer jobs at the local supermarket. I later found out they were fired for consistent tardiness. Couldn't get to work on time? What was going on? A lot, it turns out, and mostly all night long. Finally, they gave it up and went to Bill's summer house for the last few weeks of vacation. Before school started, Drew, in response to my concerns, said, "It's good for me. I've always been such a straight arrow. I'm developing my renegade side. That's what college is for, to help me learn to think for myself, to find and flesh out the rough edges."

I wasn't buying it, but then his paternal grandmother, always a lady, said, "It's great. He needs to have fun and be carefree. He's always been such a responsible child, and he's still so kind. He deserves this."

My friend Nicky agreed: "Just be glad this didn't start when he was fourteen," her voice heavy with experience. She was right. Besides, Drew was nearly grown, and my influence on such matters was waning. I was relieved when, once back at school, he balanced social life and serious study. Yet by the end of his junior year he had no energy for the former and little for the latter. Had I known, I would have longed for that renegade, tanned nineteen-year-old who romped his way through a summer without a care in sight.

At spring break, still pale and congested, he seemed all right. The drugs helped, and he was reluctant to engage in health talk. One day he did discuss a delicate issue—his sexuality. Something was wrong. He didn't feel very sexual, and he found this disturbing. Did sexuality decrease over time in relationships, he asked. I didn't probe for exact details and definitions. I should have. I was vague and answered in clichés. Yes, sex changes over time; it gets deeper, perhaps less frequent, and so forth. I didn't know how extreme the situation had become, and I was reluctant to set up false "normals," insecurities. Drew still looked worried. I suggested another visit to our family doctor despite the doctor's failure on the dry-skin problem. Drew was relieved. He wanted physiological causes explored. One of his friends had required surgery to correct a penile blood vessel rupture, and this loomed large in his mind. At this time we were making no connections among headaches, dry skin, fatigue, and low sex drive.

Drew came home from the doctor's office discouraged. No answer to be had there. The doctor had listened to his concerns. After a physical check, his kindly response, "When were your last exams?" was followed by a lecture on college stress. (If there's one thing doctors want to talk about less than nutrition, it's sexuality.) Drew decided this was his last visit to the family doctor. We all agreed that Drew was stressed, but it turned out that the stress was a result of his ongoing physical miseries, not the cause.

School ended. With an honor-roll report card, what could be so wrong? Drew had stopped eating dairy products, and his headaches were better. He rarely needed the drugs, and he said he felt fine. Drew and Rebecca got jobs in Boston, both living with us for the summer. They were busy. In fact, after work Rebecca was more likely than Drew to lie on the couch exhausted. They went to movies; they went out with friends. Drew never missed a day of work. There were animated dinner-table discussions. We all had so much fun that summer.

I fixed lots of healthy foods—whole grains, fresh vegetables and fruits, fresh fish. It appeared that we all thrived. But he was *so* pale. Drew, always fair, was now ghostly. And so thin. Those were the only clues that summer, and we ignored them.

There was one other problem mentioned toward the end of the summer. Drew reported a slight double vision in his left eye when he looked to the left. "Eye strain," I said. "Never again take an eight-hour-a-day job in front of a computer," I said. "Canada has laws protecting computer workers from just these sorts of effects," I said—perhaps somewhat desperately. (Oh please, don't let there be anything more.)

Summer ended. Rebecca left for a semester to study culture and politics in Beijing, China. Drew was to be a senior. We went to the bank to get semester finances sorted out before driving to Connecticut. While waiting in line, Drew said he was tired. He went to sit on a couch. His tall, lanky body seemed to fold in on itself as he sat down. Inadvertently, I glimpsed him out of the corner of my eye. A current of dread passed through me as a vision I'd been avoiding for months flashed in front of my eyes. In one split fraction of a second I confronted this avoidance squarely, and awareness forced its way through layers of carefully secured barriers. (Once, walking through a brightly lit department store at about age forty, I had had a similar experience. The corner of my eye caught a glimpse of myself in a mirror—a face not carefully composed for its reflection. Who is that middle-aged woman? Where is the twenty-five-year-old I know myself to be? A gulp. Later I laughed at my vanity.) This time I also gulped, but I didn't laugh. Drew sat on the brocade couch, legs crossed, so thin, his clothes hanging on him. Hadn't those old green work pants plucked from some buy-by-the-bag used clothing store once fit him? Was that improbable T-shirt with the grinning surfer on the faded blue wave, underscored with a "Surfing Against Sexism" slogan, always so loose? Drew's shaggy blond hair fell into a face etched in muted pain, his color past white to translucent gray. He looked like a cancer patient or a person with AIDS. He was truly a skeleton of his former self. My eyes filled with tears. I knew as surely as he was sitting there that I had been fooling myself, blinding myself to what was plain— no, obvious. My son was seriously ill. I knew this with a certainty so strong it was more a physical reality than a conscious thought. Too late to tell him now; we were leaving for his college in thirty minutes.

On the ride back to school I casually asked Drew how he was feeling. "Fine," he said, "a bit of a headache." But he was excited about school. His friends were exuberant. They hugged and yelled, shrieked across corridors at each other, exhibited the exhausting energy of the young. I was glad I hadn't scared him with my fears, but action was needed and soon. Sooner, it turned out, than I knew.

I drove home, walked in the door, burst into tears, and told Stephen my worries. Why hadn't we looked into this during the summer? The next real chance at extended medical workups wasn't until Christmas vacation, when Drew was going to California. I called his father. "Something is wrong," I said. "Make appointments with the neurologist at Stanford for a whole new round of medical workups." Finally, after a year, I felt fierce. "I've been hiding my head in the sand," I raged. "I should have known better."

My own classes started. Drew sounded great on the phone. He was having some trouble reading but had an appointment with an ophthalmologist. "Great," I said, "he'll give you drops for the strain." I was sure my son was ill, but I saw no relation between his general decline and double vision.

On Monday, September 16, 1991, Stephen phoned me at work. Drew had called. He had seen the eye doctor. Something was wrong. He had an appointment the next day with a neurologist. I called Drew back.

In the face of small crises I can become overly nervous, but in real emergencies I'm a calm rock. This felt like an emergency. Drew, always understated, sounded less so on the phone. The ophthalmologist said he had a sixth-nerve palsy behind his eye. This might mean a virus that would cure itself, an unexplainable condition that could require temporary corrective prism glasses, Lyme's disease from a tick bite, or diabetes;

or it could mean a tumor pressing on the nerve. Drew relayed all of this in a straightforward tone that got rougher toward the end and then turned into an outpour: "I'm so sick of being sick. What's happening to my body? I can't read, I'm behind in all my classes, my professors think I'm being lazy, I'm too tired to do anything. I can't stand another problem."

I arranged to go down the next day and take him to the neurologist. I then called the eye doctor. Having been a patient and researcher, I'm sensitive to medical cues. As soon as I gave the receptionist my name, the doctor came right to the phone—most unusual. Doctors, too busy to take calls as they come in, generally call you back. Most suspicious. "Yes," he said, "I am concerned." He had talked with the neurologist, and they agreed that a complete workup was necessary, the sooner the better. Disaster: one doctor had talked to another *before* the consultation. An appointment the next day—not in two weeks, the next day. The eye doctor was very nice, too nice. He sounded sympathetic. I didn't want sympathy; I wanted reassurance. He didn't give it. I explained the situation to my department office manager, Janice, saying I wouldn't be in the next day. She, a mother, expressed concern. I remained impassive. I called Stephen and gave an official report. All went smoothly. I appeared unperturbed. But I forgot a meeting, and I couldn't remember what I'd said in my afternoon seminar. Probably not much.

I thought things were under control. After all, I'd wanted more tests, and perhaps this would solve a year of mysteries. It did.

Tuesday morning I dressed carefully; doctors are more comfortable with people with whom they can identify. In my research I'd seen many cases of doctors—sometimes unwittingly, sometimes not—treating patients differently on the basis of appearance. For example, people in jeans risked not receiving as much information as people in "appropriate" dress. I wanted to get everything I could out of this appointment. I put on my most rational academic face and dress. I ate breakfast, kissed Stephen good-bye, and set off briskly.

Five minutes from the house something unexpected happened. I started to cry. I cried across town, I cried up Route 2 and down Route 95, and two hours later I was still crying as I drove onto the off-ramp to New London. My only child. My perfect son. When he was small, my friends teasingly referred to him as "the perfect child," so shamelessly had I bragged about him.

Drew had mostly been a sunbeam. He was open and smart and handsome. Yes, he was sloppy; yes, he was forgetful; and he had a host of vague faults; but he was unfailingly kind, and he didn't deserve this. The unknown "this," that I somehow knew was serious, was a tumor somewhere in his head, a "this" that was going to be cancer. My own pessimism had leapt to the fore. Was he going to die?

I pulled into a gas station, soaked my eyes in cold water, rearranged my mind and my face, and set off for Connecticut College. First a big hug. Nothing serious going on here. We'll get to the bottom of this, all for the good, and so on. The worry on Drew's face softened. We went to his favorite restaurant and ate lots.

"No one really sick could eat as much as you do," I joked, perplexed by such a large appetite in a person who by now was emaciated. I was finally paying attention.

The neurologist looked like a Yale or Princeton man: navy blue blazer, blue-oxford cloth shirt, striped tie, khaki pants, well-shined tassel loafers, casual elegance, and a hint of aftershave, something traditional. Mostly he asked questions, medical history details. He did the standard neurological exam—eyes following finger, reflexes flexing. He seemed unperturbed. We seemed unperturbed. So civilized. He offered no information. He had no information until he saw the test results. I might as well have worn jeans. He ordered magnetic resonance imaging (MRI, a diagnostic technique that uses a high-strength magnet, radio-frequency signals, and a computer, to produce a sharper image than that of a CAT scan)* of Drew's head and extensive blood tests. I watched carefully for hints. Of the thousands of doctor-patient encounters I had observed, how often I had seen on doctor's faces previews of the devastation awaiting unsuspecting patients. I observed; I saw nothing. One clue: the MRI had to be done in the next ten days at the latest. If the local hospital was booked, try Yale, he told his secretary. The pattern of speed, so often frustratingly lacking in medicine, troubled me.

"He didn't seem too concerned," I reassured my son. "Probably you have one of those weird viruses that attacks, attacks, and then disappears," I lied.

I talked with the school nurse. I talked with Drew's dean. Here I

---

*MRI is considerably more expensive than a CAT scan. Often doctors are pressured to order a CAT scan instead of an MRI for this reason despite the more precise and thus more reliable diagnostic abilities of MRI technologies.

was more candid. "I want no pressure, I want support, I want a memo to each of his professors. He is no shirker. He may have a tumor."

Driving back to his dorm, Drew spotted friends on the way to a soccer game. So long. He thanked me for coming, gave me a hug, and ran off, the confidence of youth momentarily restored.

Now the wait. Blood work would be back by the end of the week, the MRI by the end of the following week. I can't remember whether I worried all through those days or put it out of my mind. I must have called Drew, but I have no idea what we said to each other. I know I taught my classes and caught the flu for the first time in years. I remember lying in bed and, when I could, reading thick novels from the library. Titles, authors? I have no idea. I must have talked with Stephen at length about my unexpected tears and fears on the drive to New London, but neither of us can remember. We were both numb.

On Friday, September 20, I called Dr. N's office for the blood test results. Drew had also called. Thyroid trouble. Of course. Fatigue, headaches, weight loss, dry skin: all signs of thyroid deficiency. Yes! I hugged Janice, relief flooding through me. Thyroid was easy. Lots of people had thyroid problems. A pill. So what? A pill compared to surgery, chemotherapy, radiation, hair loss, death. Nothing, I crowed to Drew, to Stephen, to the few I confided in. Thyroid—why hadn't I thought of that? It didn't explain the vision problem, but perhaps that was separate. Medication would probably be temporary. Thank God. I still had the flu, and the MRI was still to be done, but I could start breathing again.

I stayed home sick for a few days. I could take care of myself. I enjoyed lolling under a new puff. I even remember what I read.

Drew's experience was different. Yes, if it was only thyroid, that was great. In the meantime he couldn't keep his balance to dance or move athletically, his head hurt all the time, his double vision increased, he couldn't read anything or concentrate in class, and with no Rebecca, he stayed in bed more and made it to meals less. I didn't know any of this because he didn't talk about it. For me the worst was over; for Drew, it was ill as usual.

The hospital staff did the MRI on Wednesday, September 25. I called the doctor on Thursday. His secretary said he was in surgery, but he would call in the evening if he was out in time; otherwise, tomorrow. My fears flowered. I know too much. If the MRI was normal, she probably would have told me. Maybe not, I second-guessed. MRIs may be more complicated. I didn't know anything about them. Perhaps they have to be read by the doctor as well as the radiologist. Maybe there's no bottom line that says "positive" or "negative." No. I was in for renewed terror. The secretary knew I was concerned. She did nothing to reassure me. Where were those paternalistic doctors I had written so critically about, who said, "There, there"? I wanted a "there, there," and no one would give it to me.

Drew sounded worried.

"Neurosurgeons sometimes are in surgery until late hours—ten or eleven," I reassured him. "Neurosurgeries can be long and complicated," I said, fending off the encroaching fear that we might learn just how long and complicated. Only one more day. Drew sighed and laughed. I continued to be touched by his ability to be reassured by me. Isn't that what parents are all about, knowing what's best in times of trouble? No matter how much maturing had taken place, all that distancing to be a man, I was still Drew's mom; and if he told me where it hurt, I could make it better. I always had in the past—until recently, that is. But beliefs die hard. He sounded hopeful by the end of the conversation, and I took the last vestiges of my flu to bed.

By two o'clock Friday afternoon, no call. No news is good news? It didn't feel that way. I called.

"The doctor's just come in, and he's going over everything now. Please hold."

Everything? What everything?

I yelled to Stephen, who had just arrived home, to come upstairs. I said I was on hold, and I knew the news was bad.

"Ms. Todd"—an abrupt interruption in my ear—"I've got the MRI here in front of me, and there *is* a tumor."

I turned into a textbook case study of a traumatized patient as he droned on—optic nerve, aggressive, fast-growing, very large, sixth nerve, need to move quickly—I caught words, but a buzz in my head kept me from connecting them. He gave me the names of two surgeons in Boston: "There are six surgeons in the world I would let operate on my head, and two are in Boston. You're lucky."

Lucky? Later I would think we were lucky. At two fifteen on Friday September 27, I felt we were the unluckiest people in the history of the world. The doctor had a call in to Drew; so did I. We both wanted to talk to him. He wasn't in.

Of the two great surgeons in Boston, one was busy, and the other was away. I called Drew's father in California. We cried. Gotta go, gotta find a great surgeon. In my research I'd observed ill people hearing devastating news, trying to make decisions and arrange medical care, but I'd never lived it. Think, think what to do. To get good, let alone great, health care in America, you need good insurance. That was in place. You need to know how the system works and make it work for you. I knew a lot about that. You need the best doctors. The more serious and specialized the problem, the more you need the best. All doctors are not equal; few are the best. How to get to the recalcitrant best? Pull. Know someone who knows someone.

Stephen called Rebecca's father, a psychiatrist doing neuroscience research. He made some calls. Within an hour we had a meeting set up for the next day, Saturday, September 28, at 10:00 A.M., with one of the great doctors. We were getting luckier and beginning to feel it in twinges. We would pick up Drew and a copy of the MRI early Saturday morning in New London. What do people do who don't have all of this, I moaned to myself. Some get less; some get none. You don't only need money and knowledge; you need to know someone. What if Drew were uninsured or less privileged? Would he receive this level of care? In the fall of 1991 it was unlikely. The medical sociologist in me raged, the mother rejoiced. For now I could think only of Drew. Drew had money, insurance, support, and pull. Everything that could be done would be done. But a terrible fear remained. Despite his entitlement, Drew still might die of a large, fast-growing, aggressive tumor that had been repeatedly misdiagnosed and steadily debilitating him for over a year.

Drew called. Yes, he had talked to the doctor; yes, he was freaked. He sounded teary. But he was also relieved to have an explanation for a year full of questions. I presented the plan calmly and soothingly. We would pick him up at 6:30 A.M., pick up the MRI at 7:00 A.M., and be back in Boston to meet our great doctor on Saturday morning, one of his rare times off, at 10:00 A.M. We would come down and spend the night in New London if Drew wanted us to. He didn't. He spent the night with his friends, all crowded in his room, laughing and crying, comforting and talking, supporting each other in what, for many, Drew included, was a first round with that especially unpredictable part of life we North Americans fear and loathe—mortality.

At four thirty Saturday morning we left the house. For once I didn't ask Stephen to drive more slowly. For once I didn't have much to say. We arrived early, but Drew was up. He hadn't been to bed. He hugged his close friend Ian good-bye, and both cried. We went to pick up the copy of the MRI; those pieces of floppy celluloid that were having such an impact on our lives. While the technician was making copies, I did what mothers across time and cultures do for their children in times of crisis: I went in search of food. It was too early for soup—oatmeal would have to do.

Chapter Two

I'VE NEVER HEARD
THAT ONE BEFORE

ood. I'd been paying a lot of attention to food lately, probably too much. But I'd learned how to use it to heal myself; maybe it would help heal Drew. I interrupt Drew's story here to include a chapter on my own health history. This may seem an abrupt departure from the main themes of this book, and in a sense it is. This is a book about Drew's illness, not mine. It is a book about cancer, an illness I've never had. It is a story about combining the best of Western and Eastern medicines to heal illness, whereas I was helped essentially by Eastern therapies alone.

However, what I learned during my own bouts with illness taught me how to help Drew cope with his. It's difficult to learn new bodies of knowledge during a crisis. Information explodes in your face like a fast ball; decisions are made before you know they exist. You're roiled by guilt (what did I do wrong, how did I let my child get cancer?) and fear (will my child die?). Mothers I spoke with in waiting rooms about the techniques Drew was using felt inadequate because they didn't know much about alternative medicines.

"How did you find all this out?" they'd ask, self-doubt etched in their faces. No need for guilt, I quickly assured, as I explained that I had discovered Eastern techniques during an illness of my own. In fact, the strategies I used for myself in the year before Drew was diagnosed with cancer now seem merely a training ground for the really big event— Drew's recovery. Thus, in this chapter I review that training ground to make Drew's story and how I learned about the treatments he used more understandable.

My own troubled health began with a long cycle of infections and antibiotics in the late 1970s. As the medications failed, dosages and strengths were increased, but the infections prevailed. With time they abated on their own, but my immune system had been assaulted by the overprescription of powerful antibiotics and began gradually to decline (later I was to be labeled as suffering from a "compromised immune system").

I didn't wake up one day feeling sick, nor can I pinpoint the exact date I started having vague reactions to things that had never bothered me before. The decline from being healthy, when I could eat all foods and inhale routine substances (such as new paint), to being hardly able to get out of bed, diagnosed with early-stage emphysema, took fifteen years. It seemed I had developed a strange allergy to the environment around me, a puzzling illness that had no name, diagnosis, or known solution. Other people had it, but each case was different, and no one knew where it came from or what to do about it. It was variously called environmental illness (EI), multiple chemical sensitivities, candidiasis, or a compromised immune system; before more was known about it, some denied that it existed at all, labeling it depression.

Having grown up in the last years of optimism, the science-knows-all 1950s, despite all the skepticism of the succeeding decades as well as my training as a critical medical sociologist, I was not prepared for the ignorance and lack of scientific knowledge I now faced. Where were the tests and the pills that would make this go away? By late 1990, deeply fatigued but unable to sleep, allergic to the foods, scents, and chemicals that pervade daily life, with lungs that I'd never noticed before now barely functioning, I longed for a quick fix or any fix at all. How had I become so sick?

No one seemed to have any answers. For ten years I had tried dreadful diets and medications galore to help my growing allergies, and I did get better. With time this disease with no name became a background noise that was mostly a nuisance. It didn't interfere with my life most of the time. Then, in the late 1980s, it got much worse.

In 1988, Stephen and I bought an old Victorian house and had the first floor completely renovated. With the last coat of polyurethane drying on the kitchen cabinets, we moved in. After a few months I sometimes noticed having trouble taking a full breath. My sleep became fragmented. Moreover, my allergies were increasingly bothersome. I didn't yet connect my increased sensitivities to the new paint, varnishes, carpets, and particle boards that were installed in this renovation. Moving into the house with an already compromised immune system, these chemicals added the finishing touch.

In the fall of 1990, while Drew was in Washington suffering sinus pain and fatigue, I was in Boston having difficulty breathing. Two of my classes were in renovated classrooms with newly installed carpets. In 1987 and 1988, the Environmental Protection Agency (EPA) installed new carpeting in its Washington offices. Because so many of the staff became ill, it was removed and replaced with tiles. Following this incident and others, Rosalind Anderson of Anderson Laboratories conducted studies on mice confined with chemicals found in carpeting. She reported severe neurological damage and even death in the mice.[1] In 1993, despite a history of disclaimers regarding risks from new carpets, manufacturers bowed to a congressional nudge to attach warning labels to new carpets, alerting buyers to possible harmful effects from chemicals.[2] But I didn't know any of this in 1990. I did, however, begin to connect breathing troubles, allergic reactions, and insomnia with the days I taught in those newly carpeted rooms. But mostly I failed to make connections, just as I later failed to make connections among Drew's complaints. If I didn't pay much attention, maybe the pain would go away. If I looked it straight in the eye, no telling what I'd see.

In the fall of 1990, the *New York Times* published an article on environmental illness, newly labeled "sick building syndrome." It seemed some people were sensitive to the increasing chemicalization of society—chemicals in building materials, foods, upholstery, the myriad objects of daily life. Some of these ill people were living in specially designed allergy-free ceramic trailers in Texas, unable to be around anyone or anything. Although I too-adamantly dismissed such a possibility for myself, I did seek out a doctor trained in environmental medicine. She did tests—blood and skin—for levels of formaldehyde, one of the most common chemicals causing problems. The results of both were high enough to pickle me. Wasn't formaldehyde something frogs and cadavers were stored in? I hadn't realized that it surrounded me as pervasively as the air I breathed, especially in the materials in a newly renovated house. What to do? Two approaches were advised: first, try to strengthen myself, diminishing my sensitivities; second, try to de-chemicalize my environment—not a simple task.

Out with our wonderfully comfortable new mattress. Most new mattresses, it turns out, have enough chemicals in them to be pure poison. I found mail order catalogs specializing in untreated products. All conventional bedding is laced with formaldehyde; most cleaning products are toxic; clothing is finished with an endless array of toxins. Did I want to know this? I did not. Did I need the information that dioxin, a deadly chemical, is in tampons and paper products? Formal-dehyde was a listed ingredient in my shampoo, and pesticides pervade what we eat, wear, and breathe, not to mention the chemicals in dry-cleaning fluids, leather goods, cosmetics, and food. Food. Where to begin? There seemed no end. Around three thousand chemicals, many shown—or suspected—to cause cancer, have entered our foods.

Take the all-American beverage, milk, one of the Food and Drug Administration's most regulated foods. Cows may legally be fed eighty-two drugs, as well as an assortment of veterinary drugs unregulated by the FDA; cows also ingest pesticides from feed. There are roughly sixty cancer-linked pesticides, currently allowed by the EPA, in use in our food supply.

Residues in milk have caused concern: they are connected to allergic reactions, to stronger bacteria grown more resistant in response to anti-biotics, and to possible cancer risks. Interestingly, a 1990 study of twenty-eight countries found breast cancer on the increase in all except one—Israel. The scientists had expected the increase to be universal. On close examination, the only notable change they found that might ac-count for the decrease in Israel was the banning of three carcinogenic pesticides found in milk. The FDA is working to improve regulations of this food that they already regulate more than most other foods, but so far they are required to test for only four of the drugs, ignoring the possibility of pesticides.[3] With the pesticides and fertilizers used in agri-culture, the hormones fed to livestock, and the preservatives, colorings, and processing agents used in food preparation, the surprise isn't that I got sick but that any of us are well. Even if most people do not react immediately to these toxins as I did, shouldn't we be looking at the pervasive use of known carcinogenic chemicals and the disturbing rise in American cancer rates?

Even more troubling was the information I came across on how children's toys are made. Toy stores are filled with products made of vinyl plastic, which includes vinyl chloride, polyvinyl chloride (PVC), and polyvinylpyrrolidone (PVP). Both PVC and PVP are considered carcinogenic. PVC emits vinyl chloride, a pollutant on the EPA's priority list of substances hazardous to human health. Since the EPA is widely criticized for being slow to act on or label dangerous pollutants, when they say something's hazardous and a priority, I say, pay attention. PVP, a carcinogen, causes lung disease and is dangerous enough for NASA to have removed it from use in space capsules. NASA too is not known for its environmental consciousness. It is thus with sadness that I read in Nancy Sokol Green's book, *Poisoning Our Children: Surviving in a Toxic World*, that even as she recovers from environmental illness herself, becoming less sensitive to most chemicals, she still cannot go into toy stores without becoming sick—they are too hazardous to her health.[4]

A common response to such information overload is "Oh, everything causes cancer; I can't worry about everything." I sympathize. My mind said no, this is not possible, but my body said I had to pay attention; it gave me no choice. In fact none of us has a choice if we want a healthier society.

I started reading—my first approach to everything. But reading the newspaper, books, and magazines made my lungs react. In fifteen minutes I would be gasping for air. The doctor said I was reacting to the petrochemicals and leads in the inks and perhaps the glues in the book bindings as well. Stop reading for a while, she suggested.

I did what she recommended, but cures remained elusive. What works for one person has no effect on others. Thus, while some achieve good health, or degrees of it, the road is long and paved with discarded remedies.

We who suffer from these mysterious reactions are all ahead of our time. We live in a society that asks a lot of everybody. The environment is hazardous to everyone's health: much of our food, even fresh food, is a chemical feast; our medical treatments can harm the body as well as help it; new stronger bacteria and viruses plague us; and our fluctuating economy, despite reform, is making it harder to address these problems.

Immune dysfunction in the face of all of this shows up in increased cancer rates, in a host of immune system diseases—AIDS, herpes, lupus, multiple sclerosis (MS), for example—and in those of us who become overly sensitive to the world around us. Some equate us with canaries sent down to test the air in mine shafts—the harbingers of bad news, predictors of the future. People with a dysfunctional immunity may show a mirror image of an increasingly dysfunctional social and natural environment.

My conventional family doctor, the same one who later told Drew his headaches were college stress, dismissed the diagnosis of environmental illness or chemical sensitivities and ordered a chest X ray. He'd always been sympathetic and had never treated me as if I were crazy, but he disagreed with these "fads," as he called them. He wanted proof. There was none. He had always acknowledged the legitimacy of my problems, but he, like so many others, didn't know what they were or what to do about them.

Controversy rages about environmental illness. Conventional medicine, holding onto what it knows, wants one set of causes with one set of symptoms, generalizable to all patients, and a scientifically proven cure. None of the above fits here. EI has multiple causes, different symptoms in each case, and no known cure. Modern medicine, facing more unknowns and incurables, clings to the notion of "scientific proof" as a basis for medical practice. But the fact is that mainstream medicine, while claiming this cloak of scientific legitimacy, is full of treatments that are little understood or "proven." In 1979, researchers reported in the *New England Journal of Medicine* that over the past thirty years, fewer than 5 percent of studies published in major medical journals had been based on randomized, controlled trials. Over this time span the frequency of weak research designs increased.[5] Good evidence from well-executed studies is important and does exist, just not as much as we think.

I didn't really blame doctors for wanting nothing to do with my illness. I understood all too well; I didn't want anything to do with it either. If I were ever to feel well, however, I had to search for answers. Medical literature at that time identified the cause as depression, a common label when no one knows what's going on. Depression! Of course I was depressed. I could hardly breathe, I seldom slept yet was too tired to get out of bed and I'd had to replace many of my belongings. Only a complete fool wouldn't be depressed. But like my son's stress, my depression was a result of illness, not its cause. (Today EI is being taken more seriously as a physiological, immune system–related problem.)

The chest X ray results came back. Now I was legitimate. No longer was I someone with vague complaints that changed too often and came and went a bit too capriciously over the years to be taken very seriously. Now there was an X ray, a piece of celluloid showing an inflammation in the lung. Early-stage emphysema, the radiologist said.

How could someone my age who didn't smoke or live with smokers have emphysema? The experts pondered.

"Formaldehyde," I said. "I'm sensitive to it," I reminded. "I haven't been able to breathe properly since being exposed to it," I offered. Plunging on, "CNN says workers who make particle-board products in New Mexico are coughing up blood and contracting lung disease at an alarming rate," I babbled. "In England, doctors are having people do intense breathing in clean air for lung problems and producing interesting results," I offered with one last gasp.

"Hummm," intoned the bored physician, as though listening to the lunatic fringe. "I've never heard that one before."

"Then what?" I asked. After all, I'd spent forty-four years with great lungs before my own chemical exposure.

"I don't know. We'll follow up in six months."

"What do you suggest I do to make my lungs better?"

"Take it easy, when you can. There's really nothing to do here. Emphysema isn't reversible."

Great. Go home, lie around, and try to breathe. Perhaps a respirator would help. I had given conventional medicine its best shot. Although Western medicine was to save Drew's life, it was alternative,* more Eastern treatments that would help me.

---

*Ever since allopathic (conventional) medicine took control of U.S. health care (a process that culminated in this century), all other methods—for example, Eastern medical practices and homeopathy—have been lumped together as "alternatives" and largely dismissed. These other methods, however, have not always been considered alternatives in this country (in the nineteenth century, for example, homeopathy flourished in the United States) or in others (homeopathic medicine exists alongside allopathic medicine in England; in China, acupuncture has been a mainstream healing method for several thousand years). The use of the label "alternative" for the Eastern methods used in this book is thus historically and culturally specific to modern U.S. usage. For information on the history of the rise of allopathic medicine and the exclusion of all other models, see Paul Starr (New York: Basic Books, 1982), *The Social Transformation of American Medicine*; Barbara Ehrenreich and Deirdre English (Garden City, N.Y.: Anchor Books, 1978), *For Her Own Good: 150 Years of the Experts' Advice to Women*; Rosemary Stevens (New Haven: Yale University Press, 1971), *American Medicine and the Public Interest*.

Three alternatives opened up, or perhaps I was now able to see what had been there all along.

First, I went to an acupuncturist to strengthen my system. The treatments primarily increased my energy.

Second, a yoga teacher, Karin, started coaching me on deep breathing exercises; some of the positions were upside down, inverted so that oxygen and blood would rush to my lungs, enlarging and healing them. I could feel it helping.

Third, and most important, I made dietary changes, but these took longer for me to try. I am five feet seven inches tall; by the winter of 1990 I weighed a hundred pounds. Although I was eating regularly, my body was not benefiting much, and I'd lost fifteen pounds in several months. Drew came home for Christmas vacation fatigued and suffering from a chronic headache. Despite his own pain, he was shocked at how ill I looked. He urged me to look further for a cure. Karin suggested macrobiotics, a healing, natural-foods diet, as a way to detoxify my system and start repairing the damage done to my body. Only then would I start absorbing nutrients.

Macrobiotics. Wasn't that just eating brown rice or joining a cult? I'd tried many restrictive diets, but this was too much. Besides, the use of soy sauce and other fermented foods would trigger my mold allergies, making me sicker. I was polite but uninterested. Besides, the few people I'd ever seen who ate this way all looked pale, too thin, and unhealthy to me. Somehow, I didn't register that Karin, at forty-nine and macrobiotic for much of her adult life, was the opposite of this stereotype. Radiant and youthful in looks and energy, she was a walking advertisement for balanced diet and exercise.

I did the acupuncture and yoga faithfully and I did feel better. But I was failing to thrive, and my food allergies became increasingly severe.

Life, like my body, was becoming uncomfortably slim. I moved my classes to older, uncarpeted rooms, but the Xerox machine near my office bothered me. I spent less and less time at work, more and more time in bed. It's difficult to be a college professor and not be able to read. Enclosed public places such as movie houses, theaters, and concert and lecture halls were mainly off-limits because the carpeting, synthetic seats, and perfumed patrons overwhelmed me, leaving my lungs struggling for air, my nights sleepless, and an itch under my skin. The itch, I thought, must be what DTs feel like, a toxic reaction that manifests in what I came to picture as army ants crawling rapidly around inside me, just under the surface.

I couldn't go anywhere. I couldn't read; most food made me sick; my career as a researcher had come to a standstill. Macrobiotics? What is that anyway? Maybe my reluctance had been hasty. It seemed as though it was macrobiotics or the ceramic trailer in Texas. Stephen and Drew urged the former remedy.

Sherry Rogers, a doctor in Syracuse, New York, specializes in environmental medicine. She herself had been much sicker than I from chemical sensitivities, impossible as that seemed to me. She had come back from her bed fully cured, to write a series of books on the subject and maintain a thriving practice helping others with this strange illness. I ordered the books that I couldn't read. They were printed in Syracuse and had to be mailed from the printer. I can only assume that she wrote them primarily for her patients. I literally stumbled upon an order form, for no one I talked with, even those who had heard of her, knew anything about her books. They did not look impressive: poorly edited, with scanty indexes, the typeset looked typed even in this age of computers, and printed in terribly toxic ink. Not an auspicious beginning. But I started with the how-to book.

You Are What You Ate: A Macrobiotic Way, smelly ink and all, made me sick while reading it but in effect threw me a lifeline. My approach to EI had been one of searching for outside cures. I was willing to be active, to work hard, and, in fact, to stand on my head to affect this cure, but I expected physicians to provide at least the framework for the solution. That approach works well for acute disease—a strep throat, appendicitis, even some forms of cancer, as I was all too soon to learn—but it didn't work for EI. Here, large amounts of a toxic substance(s) first make you ill. Once you are sensitive, small amounts can trigger the reaction. These small amounts are everywhere, so you are constantly ill. There is no quick way to break this cycle. In my heart of hearts, despite all my research on the inability of the acute medical model to help many, particularly chronic diseases, I wanted that speedy help. Sherry Rogers's book reminded me that that wasn't going to happen. She claimed that my body could heal itself if given some encouragement, and she told me how.

Stephen, a continuing and worried support, set off for the health food store with a list of foods we had never heard of. We pored over the strange ingredients: different dark and dangerous-looking seaweeds (full of vitamins and minerals); lots of leafy greens and round, sweet root vegetables; strange grains, like quinoa and brown rice in various lengths; seeds such as sesame and pumpkin. These were mostly organic and all fresh.

I bravely set out to try some of the book's suggestions. To start, during the acute healing phase, proportions are important (50–60% grains, 20–30% greens, 5–10% beans, 5–10% nuts, seeds, seaweeds). Fermented foods such as tamari (soy sauce), miso soup, and the extraordinary umeboshi plum would come later, when I was healthier.

Day 1 soup. I chopped, grated, and rinsed, mixing squash, seaweed, onion, and rice, adding some kale at the end. It was without a doubt the most revolting food I had ever eaten. Better to die, I wailed, than eat this. It smelled like low tide on a humid day and tasted worse. My sense of humor, increasingly strained, abandoned me. I went back to bed.

Stephen read the book. "There are lots of other ways you can eat this food," he reassured me.

Neither of us had any idea if nutrition would work, but we both felt out of options. Back to the stove. Soft, short-grain brown rice, topped with crumbled, crunchy wakame seaweed, finely chopped green onions, and parsley. Lightly steamed carrots with sesame seeds. Baked sweet winter squash stuffed with millet, minced onion, roasted sunflower seeds, and a touch of grated fresh ginger. Great—this I could eat. And eat it I did, for about ten days. I tentatively admitted to feeling a bit better. No need for a leap into optimism, but I was sleeping better, my breathing was more even, and the army ants were more sluggish. I now had the energy to investigate these foods further. When Drew came home for spring break, we compared health notes. I was better; he was worse.

My kitchen became an experimental laboratory. As my energy increased, so did the variety in my cooking. Along with eating many familiar foods, such as grilled fish, sourdough bread, most vegetables and salads, I discovered a multitude of new foods: diverse vegetables— leafy broccoli rabe, rutabaga, burdock, and lotus roots; beans—anasazi, black soy, aduki; grains—yellow millet, sweet brown rice cooked with chestnuts, amaranth; novel seasonings such as tikka, gamashio, nori flakes, and so on. To my amazement I liked this food. If I balanced the foods—acid and alkaline, expansive and contractive, just as Sherry Rogers suggested—I rarely had food cravings. And to think I had considered this a restrictive diet; it was in some ways the most varied diet

I'd ever eaten, particularly in recent years as my food tolerances had narrowed.

The good news was in my slow but steady improvements. Discouraging, however, was a continuous hypersensitivity to the world around me. I needed to know more about what I was doing. But I still had trouble reading. I decided one way to learn more was to go to the Kushi Institute at Becket in western Massachusetts. Michio Kushi, the popularizer of George Ohsawa's macrobiotic theories on food and health, had first come to the United States from Japan in 1949. He enrolled at Columbia University for graduate study in his field of international law, not nutrition; but he and his wife, Aveline, began introducing the idea of whole, fresh foods, based on both a traditional Japanese diet and Ohsawa's work. Kushi's road from international law to macrobiotics is its own story, but he never looked back. Today, in their late sixties, he and Aveline travel and lecture all over the world from their base in Becket. People can come for weekend, week- or monthlong workshops to improve their own health or to learn to counsel others.

It seemed daring to venture to an unknown place, unknown in terms of environmental hazards as well as potential philosophical eccentricity. Once I'd ascertained I could have a room of my own, however, with no carpets and with a mattress that was probably circa World War II, I set off for a week's session. If nothing else, a week of fresh mountain air would be good for my lungs. If appalled by the people or the lectures, I could go for long walks and hide in my room. So suspicious. All of my skeptical armor in place, I was immediately disarmed. The staff, clear-eyed and direct, were friendly and helpful. The Kushis were away on tour, but senior counselors would be our guides. The house and grounds could use some redoing, but I wasn't complaining—no pesticides on that lawn, no fresh paint to be found.

Most interesting were the other guests. Many were seriously ill whether they looked it or not. A man in his thirties recovering from brain surgery admitted this was going to be a challenge—he, his wife, and kids went out for pizza every Saturday night. A retired dentist from South Carolina with pancreatic cancer couldn't imagine not eating ribs. His doctor had done all he could—surgery and radiation. When asked if there wasn't anything else, the doctor responded that he had heard of macrobiotics helping with terminal cancer. He didn't know anything about it, but maybe it would help. With a little investigation the dentist started the diet at home. A bit thin but otherwise healthy-looking and feeling great, he was here to learn more. The list went on: diabetes, breast cancer, fibroids, and so on. Some people had come with their healthy spouses so that they could learn together, particularly those who would need help. There were fifteen of us, and to my amazement I was the most experienced with the diet. People kept looking to me for information. I had met the wild kook at the Kushi Institute and it was me.

The days started with a gently energizing Asian exercise routine called Do-In. We tapped our bodies along energy (acupressure) points and stretched. Each day included three enormous buffet meals of creatively combined vegetables, beans, grains, and soups and a cooking class to teach us how to fix these meals. The food was lovely to look at and delicious to eat. Even the pizza lovers were enthusiastic. Each day also included a lecture on the fundamentals of macrobiotics. When I saw the schedule, I decided to go to the first lecture and skip the rest. It would be a good time to walk and breathe the fresh air. But again, my determined skepticism gave way to fascination. The sociologist in me kept me coming back. Argument was encouraged. Discussions flared, people debated and disagreed, everyone was engaged. Unable to read or spend much time at work, I delighted in the stimulation. And none of the institute's regimens or environs made me sick. The air was clean and the household environmentally protective of the land around it and thus of visitors.

The lectures, given by different people, focused on Eastern philosophies of harmony and balance. If you had these in your diet, you would have them in your being. If you had them in your being, there would be more harmony in the world. One peaceful world, the Kushi's new goal, could become a reality. At times this sequence seemed too easy. I, like others, remained skeptical of aspects of the philosophy. Our skepticism made for interesting debates, and open discussion was part of the educational atmosphere.

Other lectures emphasized a holistic view of mind connected to body, people connected to the universe. One of the lecturers quoted Carl Jung's comparison of Chinese and Western worldviews: "While the Western mind carefully sifts, weighs, selects, classifies, isolates, the Chinese picture of the moment encompasses everything down to the minutest nonsensical detail because all the ingredients make up the observed moment."[6] Whereas in the West we fragment to understand the part, the East never loses sight of the whole.

We learned the importance of chewing well when you switch to a

diet of complex carbohydrates. Careful chewing of all foods is important. But the enzymes that digest animal products are in the stomach.
Primary enzymes for digesting grains and beans, however, are in the
mouth; digestion of these foods starts with the saliva. So we spent a fair
amount of time grinding away. We learned about food ratios, the importance of sea vegetables for minerals and vitamins. Vegetarians who do
not eat sea weeds risk anemia, low B_{12}, and so forth. I was getting what I
needed—the whys for what I was already doing.

I never did take those long walks, and I went to my room only to
sleep. I made friends, especially with an academic woman struggling
with multiple allergies and diabetes. For such a sick group, spirits and
energy were high. I left with a strong sense of what I wanted to accept
and what to reject. Nobody at the institute tried to change that. The
counselors, like all good educators, wanted to open your mind, get you
to think for yourself, take the knowledge and make your own decisions.

On my return to Boston, I signed up for a macrobiotic cooking
class. The first meeting continued to debunk my stereotypic assumptions
about vegetarians. Except for Karin, I still harbored suspicions about
those who ate this diet by choice—zealots sitting around counting rice
grains, I thought, looking self-righteous and telling you denial was spiri-
tual. Where did I get these ideas?

Lots of places, I realized. The media treat people who think about
food, especially macrobiotics, with humor and suspicion. Take the popular movie *Green Card*, starring Andie McDowell and Gerard Depardieu.
Andie's boyfriend, a vegetarian, is spindly, petulant, whiny, and self-
righteous. He is also an environmentalist, usually a dubious sign on
celluloid. Gerard Depardieu, pure prime beef—increasingly so in fact—
and somewhat of a slob, just this side of picking his nose and belching,
saves Andie from the Spartan life, winning her love with fat foods and
devotion to self-indulgence. Message: real meat equals real men equals
getting the girl. Women in film fare even worse. Dr. Greerson (Diane
Wiest) in *Little Man Tate* is intellectual, successful, considered brilliant;
so in Hollywood terms she is also lonely, unable to connect to other
people, difficult, and arrogant. First we don't like her much; then,
worse, we pity her. But mostly we pity her young student, Fred, who is
taken off his customary diet, rich in Cokes, by this uptight woman and
given a brownish-green, revolting-looking blenderized health shake. Dr.
Greerson instructs: "It's not your mother's fault. Most parents are igno-
rant of the benefits of macrobiotics."

The brave Fred, braver than any of us would be, takes a gulp. Our stomachs tighten at the sight. As politely as possible, Fred throws up on the floor. Who wouldn't?

The audience doesn't pity Sophie in the film *Eating*. We just dislike her. She is macrobiotic, neurotic, and every other "otic" imaginable. She preaches to her friends, orders in a vegetarian meal for herself at a lavish buffet brimming with fresh vegetables, moralistically picks at the food, makes herself vomit afterward so that she won't gain weight, calls her therapist, bemoans her singleness, and tries to ruin everyone else's love life. It's not clear whether she's macrobiotic because she's so neurotic or neurotic because she's macrobiotic. In any case the message is clear: those who eat macrobiotic foods are lonely, borderline crazy people, and worst of all, they ruin any party.

Moralistic macrobiotic people do exist—I've met a few—but my experience has generally been the opposite. At my first cooking class, Evelyne, a petite Morrocan/French woman with the shiniest long black hair I'd ever seen, spoke to the students in a soft, comforting French accent about the foods she was preparing. She aimed to Americanize the Japanese version of macrobiotics. Sitting, taking notes were about ten men and women: an architect, a designer, two college students, a composer for Hollywood films, a business executive, a well-dressed housewife. Interesting people. Some were or had been sick; others just wanted to stay healthy. The housewife diagnosed with terminal cancer claimed macrobiotics had cured her. The composer, when told she needed a hysterectomy due to a tumor, chose another route—diet—and the tumor was gone, her uterus in place. The students were sick of dormitory food. They felt everything served was exactly what the heart and cancer associations were saying killed us. They wanted to cook for themselves. If only Drew were this interested, I thought wistfully.

Evelyne fixed a delectable meal, giving us careful instructions on cooking and the healing properties of the foods and food combinations. We then ate, talked, laughed. I hadn't done that in a while. I came home hyperbolic. Even Stephen would like these dishes. Maybe Drew would try them and feel better.

Thus, I embraced a new way of learning, by doing rather than reading; talking with people, attending lectures and classes. My critical-thinking education didn't abandon me. When no one could explain to me why yams, one of my favorite foods, were unhealthy, I continued eating and loving them. When I was told miso fermented soup was what

I needed, I wasn't ready to try it. When it became clear that some aspects of the philosophy didn't appeal to me, I ignored them. As with Sherry Rogers's terrible soup, I had to make my own choices here. But I now had the energy to make decisions. I was getting better.

As I get healthier, it seems impossible I was ever so sensitive to my environment. Was I crazy? I was luckier than most. My husband, son, extended family, in-laws, work colleagues, and friends generally treated me as a sane person caught in an insane trap. Years of knowing me as a rational person bolstered their belief that I was truly ill. After all, if tree pollen makes some people sick, why shouldn't formaldehyde? Dioxin? Benzene? Petrochemicals? Not everyone, however, is treated as respectfully as I was or has the means to pursue the remedies I discovered.

A contractor, not as lucky as I, told me he'd become ill with EI when his antichemical mask failed while he was installing Formica onto cabinet bases in a kitchen he was remodeling. He could smell the adhesive's chemicals, so he knew something was wrong, but he never suspected the devastation that would result. He had wanted to get the job finished. The result: temporary paralysis, chronic fatigue, neurological damage, in time his business and savings gone. Four years later, when I met him, he was much better but still tired easily, suffering tingling and pain in his extremities, and he was in financial debt. The incredible part of the story was that despite the adhesive's stated warnings of possible neurological and brain damage from fumes if not used properly, his doctors and family didn't believe the connection. His family eventually came around, offering him some emotional and financial support. His doctors never did. But mainly because of dietary changes, he too was recovering.

By the summer of 1991, I was getting well, and Drew was feeling better than he had in Washington. He still, however, got headaches and was thin and pale. I thought I could make him better. I tried to interest him in all the new foods I was eating. He was polite. He was relieved that it was helping me. He was happy that I loved the food. But he didn't. Drew liked the rice and beans but disliked all those vegetables. He had always been a picky eater. (As a baby he wouldn't eat the skins of hot dogs. He found a way to peel them in his mouth at age one and a half.) Seaweed? Forget it. But it was just the foods I'd grown to love that he would learn to tolerate. It was just this diet that would help him to survive his ordeal as it had helped me to survive mine.

Chapter Three

AND PLEASE, NO MORE
ONE PERCENT ODDS

*Rage is the psyche's first defense against overwhelming disaster. Fate
is unfair and man finds unfairness of such magnitude incomprehensible.*
— GERDA LERNER

We met Dr. S in the lobby of the hospital in Boston, having
driven up from Connecticut. He shook our hands, smiling just enough
to convey warmth but avoiding inappropriate cheer. His very presence
reassured us: the craggy face with thick, graying eyebrows and careful
eyes, the tweed jacket—everything soft, casual but not too casual. He
had a measured manner that proclaimed, "What we have here is serious,
but we see it all the time. We can make it go away." We clung to his eyes,
his words, his every gesture. This was one of the six neurosurgeons in the
world worthy of operating on another neurosurgeon. We would have
kissed his feet had that been required. It wasn't. Just as doctors shunned
the vagueness of my slippery ailments, they were to embrace Drew's
measurable, definable tumor. They didn't know the cause, but they
knew all about the cure. Once in his office, Dr. S began to explain: "This
sort of tumor is not uncommon. Most likely it is a benign [noncan-
cerous] pituitary tumor, which would account for the lack of hormones." The dry skin, loss of weight, fatigue, lack of sex drive—all
connected.

"It's become quite large—see here." (We craned forward to get a closer look at the MRI images, this new vision of Drew's head.) "It's pressing on your optic nerve, affecting your vision." Dr. S talked to Drew directly, including Stephen and me with his glance. He exuded confidence, confidence in the situation—not nearly as bad as the young girl he'd seen yesterday with the embolism—and confidence in himself, the great fixer. Routine. Drew had an everyday sort of tumor. We basked in Dr. S's skillful manner, his comforting assurances, his detailed explanations. He listened carefully to all of our questions, giving us the hoped-for answers to each.

The schedule would be hectic. The tumor, having grown quickly, was larger than he expected. Yes, it must come out immediately, before it caused more vision trouble or grew to be inoperable. The schedule: doctors' appointments this coming week, surgery the following week. Monday, the neuroradiologists (the best in the world, we were told) would examine the MRI, and on their recommendations we would proceed.

We felt better. Dr. S had told it to us straight but smooth, the iron fist in a velvet glove. We were grateful for that velvet glove. The ride home from the hospital was nearly a celebration. What a long way to have come in under twenty-four hours. It was a tumor, it was a nightmare, but it was common, it was benign, it would be over soon. Home to bed. After a few phone calls, a few tears, we spent the afternoon asleep.

I don't remember much about Sunday. Drew was sicker than when I had last seen him. No longer having to pretend wellness to himself and others, he collapsed. He mostly slept. I mostly talked on the phone. A year of reticence, avoiding talk about my own health, changed dramatically. I talked and talked, ruining the day for a multitude of friends and family. Perhaps turning horror into ritual through repeated tellings made the unreal more real, the remote more tangible.

Monday I remember well. "I'll go in and teach today and arrange substitutes for the next two weeks," I told everyone. I felt strong, a rock that Drew could lean on, and able to navigate the medical monoliths, which are trickier than most people realize. A continuous buzz of list making went through my head; clearing my desk was making the loudest noise. I set off full of purpose. I had a class to teach. My department colleagues knew the situation, but students and the general community at my university did not. Good. I could breeze through without explanations. In and out.

I got into an elevator crammed with students but missed my floor. How had that happened? Agnes from the government department got on at the twelfth floor. Were we going down?

"Hi Alexandra, how's it going?" I couldn't speak. "Just tell her fine and get off the elevator," I commanded myself. I couldn't move, couldn't answer. "That bad, huh?" laughed Agnes. I started to cry. Tears silently rolled down my cheeks, in public, on an elevator, in front of students. I was usually a hard cry in or out of public view. No longer. Agnes took my arm and led me to my office. I couldn't talk. Janice, the office manager, took over, as she was to do repeatedly in the coming months. I sat in my office, joined by Ann, the professor across the hall, and in front of this small group of sympathizers, all mothers, I sobbed. My class was to begin in ten minutes. Ann combined her class with mine, and I, crying openly, cleared my desk.

Stephen phoned to report that Dr. S had called. He had arranged appointments with various specialists for Tuesday and Wednesday; Drew was on a waiting list for surgery on Thursday. Thursday? What about next week?

"That means the best neuroradiologists in the world didn't like what they saw. That means it may not be an everyday tumor. That means time is ever more important," I said to Stephen. That means he may die, I moaned to myself. I had to get home.

I washed my face and set off, pouring out the whole story, at least tearlessly, to a professional acquaintance of Stephen's I barely know whom I met on the subway. Where was that stiff upper lip, the British detachment I had been so criticized for and was so critical of in the 1960s but had come to rely on? I found that when Drew was around, when he needed me, my background served me well. That steady composure, however, crumbled in his absence.

Everything was happening too quickly, with no time to prepare. We found ourselves on a careening conveyor belt. There seemed to be no choices here. In my medical sociology classes I cite studies that show the importance of exploring options: Is the surgery really necessary? Should it be the first line of defense or the last? Surgery rates continue to rise in the United States. Many operations are unnecessary, to the point that insurance companies may require second opinions before consenting to cover costs. How could we arrange for a second opinion, for a literature review of head tumors at the medical library? How could we agree to allow Drew's head and brain to be invaded with so little knowledge? It's not healthy to be so powerless, so passive.

In the last decade I had explored alternative approaches to health and illness, for myself and for teaching. Societies think about and treat the body in such richly diverse ways. I needed time to find out if some of the Eastern techniques I had researched could help here—not to replace Western medicine, the crisis was too immediate, but to bolster and complement what the surgeons had to offer. Was it possible to learn enough in so short a time? None of my research or personal experience involved cancer or the brain. But I did have knowledge about alternative medicines to draw on—my own, my students', and my family's.

About fifteen years ago my mother, an active seventy-year old widow, developed arthritis in her shoulder. It hurt to raise her arm; she had trouble with back zippers, reaching up to wash her hair, making the head twists necessary to drive safely. Her independent way of life was jeopardized.

"Is this the beginning of old age and all its attendant infirmities?" she asked in a brave but sad phone call. Her doctor suggested aspirin at regular intervals. It had no effect on her shoulder but caused new troubles—stomach problems. She saw a doctor talking about acupuncture on a television talk show. Acupuncture? We had all heard of it but knew nothing more. She talked with friends and decided it couldn't hurt her. We discussed it skeptically. As the pain grew more debilitating, however, what had she to lose? She called the TV station and tracked down the speaker. He was a conventional doctor and author, since become quite famous, who had also trained in acupuncture. Within three treatments she was better, and in three months the pain was gone—permanently. On the basis of this happy ending I had started researching acupuncture and Chinese medicine. What I found was impressive.

Valerie, an acupuncturist who had helped me during the past year by using pressure points and needles to detoxify my body and stimulate my immune system, squeezed Drew in on that terrible Monday afternoon. She didn't want to start treatment until after the surgery. Acupuncture works on energies in the body. Val didn't want to stimulate those energies when the tumor was so large. But she did want to talk with Drew, go over his history, check his pulses (six in each wrist, in Chinese medicine), and be ready to start treatments as soon as he returned home from the hospital. Her strategy was to strengthen his system once the surgery was over.

Drew, too tired to sit up for an hour, lay on Val's examining table. I don't know what they said, but they talked for a long time. They liked each other. Val told me later that if attitudes could cure, he would be well in a week. His wry humor, his ability to talk about what was happening, his optimism that he would come through this impressed her. In fact, Drew's sense of irony, embedded in a sunbeam nature, impressed us all. Val suggested two to three visits a week after the surgery, until he felt strong again.

Next, on Tuesday, came our first day of medical immersion. No need to worry about second opinions. By the end of the week there would be double-digit views on Drew's condition. Everyone was busy, everyone was "the best in the world," but at Dr. S's request they all made time for Drew. They didn't keep us waiting. Yes, we were lucky. In a society of historically unequal access to health care, Drew was getting the best and getting it quickly. But my heart sank. It's not that I wanted to be kept waiting or to be told, as usual, that the first available appointment was three, six, or eight weeks away. But to get such immediate treatment, Drew's had to be an "interesting case," more dangerous, perhaps rarer, than it had seemed. Without being told so, I felt sure that the neuroradiologists interpreted the MRI more seriously. Where was the "routine," the "quite common"? Long gone, apparently.

Late Tuesday afternoon, with Drew paler than ever, stooping noticeably, head pounding and vision increasingly doubled, I, with some guilt, drove him across town for one more stop. We went to see Evelyne, my cooking class teacher and a nutritional counselor. An individual consultation is essential when one is considering dietary changes. Although the nutritional framework of an anticancer diet may be generalizable, each person's illness, size, constitution, history, and so forth vary. Since some foods are medicinal, the diet must be individually tailored. (This is especially important when the ill person is a young child and quantities need to be carefully monitored.) And as with choosing any health professional, care should be taken to find a qualified, recommended person.* For example, I already knew Evelyne and her excellent reputation. Otherwise, I would have called the Kushi Institute for suggestions and asked for referrals as well as the professional backgrounds of those suggested.

Once again Drew lay down, dozing during the interview. Evelyne

---

*A caveat: Not all alternative methods or practitioners are equal. As when choosing a conventional doctor, careful research is needed. There is quackery everywhere, and the consumer needs to be careful. It is important to read up on treatments and programs, talk with people who have used different approaches and practitioners. Ask for references; if possible, do your own research or ask a friend to help you.

made detailed suggestions about what to eat and what to avoid. The healing diet for cancer is very strict, but the anecdotal evidence of its effectiveness, as well as a small but increasingly scientific data base, are exciting. For example, a Harvard School of Public Health experiment showed a later onset of induced mammary cancer in animals fed seaweed than in those not given it. The researchers' conclusion: "seaweed-fed rats had a longer time to tumor than did the control rats [19 weeks in the experimental rats versus 11 in the control group]. Seaweed has shown consistent antitumor activity in several *in vivo* animal tests."[1] Dr. Steven Rosenberg, the National Cancer Institute's chief of surgery and surgeon for Ronald Reagan's colon cancer operation, considered but decided against either radiation or chemotherapy following Reagan's surgery. Instead, he suggested a diet rich in whole grains.[2] The list goes on, including compelling case histories by survivors (see chapter 6).

The diet Evelyne advised for Drew, based on her knowledge of cancer and nutrition as well as Drew's history, was designed to give his body the most nutrients for the least work. A steak has many nutrients, but the body has to work hard to absorb them, sorting them out from fat (and in American beef, from hormones and antibiotics). Drew's body had more important work to do; his diet was going to give him even more nutrients for a fraction of the effort. (See Appendix A for a summary of Drew's diet and a list of books about healthy eating.)

Drew was polite, as usual. By now, however, he was too tired for humor, and a steak sounded just fine. The strange foods—some new even to me—and the carefully prescribed amounts overwhelmed us both. This regimen is going to be a full-time job, I thought to myself. But I clung so fiercely to this diet. Hadn't it helped me when nothing else did? I wasn't suggesting it as a replacement for medical treatment, I defended. Many people with tumors, even cancer, reject medical recommendations and just do the diet. Many unexpectedly recover. I was not advocating that, I reminded Drew, in the face of his dejected look. But when it came to miso soup with seaweed, there was no ironic humor to be found. We drove home. He's twenty-one, I reminded myself, and he has to decide for himself. It isn't fair to try to make him do this if he doesn't want to; it could make him worse in the face of such opposition.

"Think about it," I said. "It's your decision. If you want to try, I'll do all the work. If you don't, I'll understand." I think I meant it.

Drew decided to try. After all, he'd been eating this food in a slightly different form since he'd come home from Connecticut and was feeling a bit better. He'd given up dairy products the year before because they caused immediate headaches. (Evelyne thought the dairy products were causing mucus buildup in his sinus, putting pressure on the tumor and thus on his head.) After a rest, Drew's good humor returned, and we talked about the foods. He did feel overwhelmed by such a dramatic change, from dormitory food to macrobiotics. He would try it but not permanently. The new diet was a temporary aberration in his life, much like the tumor, surgery, acupuncture, obsession with the body, doctor visits, and headaches. These were temporary visitors.

Tuesday night Drew's father, Andy, arrived from California. He'd planned to come the following weekend but flew in earlier when the operation was scheduled sooner. He couldn't stand being so far away, so it was with relief that he came early. We all met at the airport with hugs and more tears. Would the tears ever stop?

Andy and I had married young, too young, when he was twenty and I was nineteen. We were two kids for the first years while Andy was in college and then graduate school. After five years we had Drew. Then we were three kids. As Andy and I grew up, we grew apart and separated when Drew was two. Although our marriage didn't last, it's unfair to say we had an unsuccessful marriage. For it was generally a time of unquestioned devotion, the last chance at feeling so secure in a world that held such promise. It is fairer to say we have had a very successful divorce, sharing parenting well and remaining friends, though at a distance. Andy and his second wife, Sally, raised Drew more than I did. We were among the first couples in California to receive joint custody. We communicated often and discussed all big decisions. No one had more parents, not to mention grandparents, than Drew—overwhelmingly so at times. But Andy and I hadn't been around each other for so many days since the divorce, and we'd never faced a real crisis with Drew. I hoped we could pull together in these unusual circumstances. Mostly we could, as it turned out.

On Wednesday, Andy, Drew, and I set off for more hospital appointments: full eye exams by a specialist in neuromedicine, then off to a memorable visit with Dr. E, an eye, ear, and sinus neurosurgeon. Dr. E was large, with an expansive manner and a broad smile. He welcomed us into his office in the manner of a host at a dinner party. After hours of medical reserve, we felt giggly in the face of such exuberance. A tumor. No need for gloom. Dr. E fairly pranced around the room, posting copies of the old CAT scan and the new MRI. We were surrounded by every possible angle of the inside of Drew's head. Dr. E grew increasingly excited as he examined the pictures. This was a man who loved his work.

"Think of this as a series of surgeries." He beamed, pointing to a celluloid blur of tumor. (Series of surgeries? Ice water trickled exquisitely down my spine, vertebra by vertebra. I kept an impassive face toward Drew as if to say, "What does he know?")

"This could be hard as stone," he said, pointing to a mass on one of the pictures. "The first surgery will go up through the nose and cut away over here and get a biopsy," he enthused. "Then we'll have to decide whether to go down through the head and see what we can get."

"Are you doing the surgery?" I interrupted, amazement in my voice.

"If appropriate. Later on, Dr. S will assess the situation, and if the tumor's spread into sinus areas, here or here"—he pointed at the pictures—"I'll be called in further down the line." He sounded thrilled, bringing to mind Melville's saw-to-leg enthusiast, Cadwallader Cuticle, MD, of whom it was said, "he would rather cut off a man's arm than dismember the wing of the most delicate pheasant."[3]

"I'd drill a neat hole right down through here"—he gently drew a small circle on the bridge of Drew's increasingly pale nose—"coming in with additional incisions here and here and maybe here." His fingers danced across Drew's face. In his medical fervor, Dr. E seemed insensitive to the fact that he was talking to and about a person.

"The tools are amazing these days," he raved. "I did exactly this surgery the other day. Very successful. Very lucky woman."

(I wondered how lucky she felt about having open-pit mining across her face.)

"Now I have to ask you both to leave while I do the exam." He bounced over to show a numb Andy and me the way out.

Could we leave this maniac alone with our son? Surely he was an impostor. It's important to like one's work, but this level of excitement, more like euphoria, over a tumor was inappropriate. Finding ourselves in the waiting room before we knew it, Andy and I looked at each other speechless. Finally, Andy asked, "What's Dr. S like?"

Dr. S. We hadn't seen him since Saturday. We still didn't know what kind of surgery he was planning. Was Drew scheduled for Thursday or still on the waiting list? It was Wednesday afternoon; shouldn't he be admitted? After numerous visits and tests, with Drew's arms bruised from one invasion after another, we stopped by Dr. S's office. His secretary had left a message with Stephen. No room on Thursday. The surgery was set for Friday. We were to check into the hospital at one o'clock on Thursday afternoon. Dr. S would come by and talk with us that evening. No, the secretary didn't know more. Dr. S wanted to talk with all the people Drew had seen before making final decisions. The surgery was two days away, and the type of surgery was still undecided. This didn't sound like an everyday pituitary tumor to me.

We went home and entertained Stephen, calming ourselves with hilarious depictions of Dr. E. For sanity's sake we turned him into a clown, someone we would never see again. Dr. S said Drew had a 99 percent chance of one surgery; one surgery it had to be, even if no one seemed to know what kind of surgery.

Wednesday night we celebrated, laughing, having fun. Here I was with my one child, my previous and current husbands, on the night before the night before surgery, having one last supper. I don't know how, but we enjoyed ourselves at a restaurant with healthy choices. Andy, curious about the nutrition plan and fully supporting it, encouraged Drew on this last night to have anything he wanted. I sat on my fears, agreed, and studied the menu. Drew, keeping his own counsel, made healthy choices. We talked and ate and nearly forgot.

Thursday at 5:00 A.M., I was wide awake. Stephen hadn't been able to sleep until 4:00 A.M., so he was impervious to my wakefulness. At 5:30 I heard Andy stirring. It seemed that one of us was wandering the house at any given hour. Drew, however, slept soundly until about 10:00 A.M.

The hospital check-in was crowded. We waited. Drew went off with Andy for more blood tests, chest X rays, an assortment of preentry procedures. We were in one of Boston's famous hospitals, a place people come to from all over the world. An international array of people waited with us. "What if in the face of all this we had to go to New Delhi for the surgery?" I wondered aloud. For every challenge we face, there is one harder, more demanding for somebody else.

Our name was called. I gathered the insurance cards, without which we would not get a foot past the entry desk. This hospital, like many large urban medical centers, has a wing for the rich and famous. I had read about it in the newspaper—rooms with a view, all to yourself, hushed quiet, brocade sofas for your visitors, pictures on the walls, a Ritz Hotel approach to healing. This was where royalty stayed, Saudi Arabian princesses with their entourage. I had scorned such indulgence. How unethical it seemed to offer such luxury in a country at a time when many were deprived of basic health services, when many, particularly the working poor, had no coverage, when many pregnant women didn't have access to prenatal care, contributing to our high infant mortality rates, especially among women and babies of color. In a country where so many have so little, why should a few have so much, especially when it comes to health care?

All true, but that was last week. A quiet room, soothing surroundings might induce faster healing and less fear in such strange surroundings.

"I want him to be in the so-called royal wing," I requested as soon as I was seated. The young admittance man surveyed his computer.

"Okay, we can put him there for an extra charge."

"Fine." Perhaps his paternal grandfather would pay. If not, I'd teach summer school. I was, at last, healthy enough to do so. Money was the last thing on my mind. I thought how lucky I was for that to be the case.

As it turned out, money didn't matter, not if you were a princess or if you were Drew. The hospital was full. Not a bed in the royal wing or the welfare ward. We waited. They found a room. It was a double room with a long-term twenty-year-old male patient they tried to keep isolated. He was indeed unfortunate: quite mentally and physically disabled, he lay bunched up, staring at the wall and periodically yelling unintelligible sounds. His chronic, odorous diarrhea required regular diaper changes day and night. Small loudspeakers by each bed kept up a steady loud and staticky calling of names to the front desk or patient rooms day and night.

This was to be a difficult night for Drew. A young, vibrant woman breezed in and introduced herself. Beth was a specialist in neurosurgery, and she was to be Drew's main nurse. "At least you have a window," she laughed. It looked out on an air shaft. We liked her. She treated Drew kindly. She treated the man in the next bed tenderly. She chatted reassuringly to Andy, Stephen, and me; she squeezed up against the side of the bed. So much for the fancy room. It's the surgery that counts, I reminded everyone over the incessant blare of the bedside loudspeaker.

A resident, the first of a long string of doctors, endocrinologists, anesthesiologists, neurosurgery residents, and neophyte medical students, came, wanting Drew's full history. We took off for a snack. When we returned, we found a youngish dark-haired man in a brown herringbone sports coat questioning Drew. He glanced dismissively at us, gave the curtain shielding the next bed an annoyed look in response to the other patient's loud groans, and pulled out a release form for Drew to sign. To my surprise he handed it to Drew. Why not to me? It was a shock to remember my baby was a man, twenty-one years old. Whoever this person was seemed to know that. He certainly had no interest in talking to the three of us.

"Before you sign this," he told Drew, "I have to tell you that with this kind of surgery, going so close to the brain and the optic nerve, there's a chance of damage—damage to the intellect part of the brain and the possibility of blindness. A more outside consequence with any surgery is death," he monotoned. "Any questions?"

What did he mean by "this kind of surgery"? Who was this man? Stephen asked him a bit coldly, suspiciously, "Who *are* you?" There was a pause and a slight turning of the head in Stephen's direction. "I'm the surgeon" was delivered briskly in response to such an inappropriate question, and no, he didn't have his cards with him. Drew asked about possibilities of more surgeries.

"Too soon to tell" was the response.

Drew signed the forms, and this man was gone before we had the wits to demand to know more. We didn't even know his name. It had happened so fast. All of the time I'd spent in hospitals doing research, observing people's bewilderment at their surroundings—how could I let this happen? If that man was the surgeon, was he a great surgeon? He looked so young. Where was Dr. S? Blindness? Brain damage? Death? What exactly were the chances here? And what about multiple surgeries? How could anyone think with that loudspeaker making so much noise?

Dr. S arrived. He soothed; he comforted. Here was the story. Drew's nostrils were too small to operate through his nose. He, Dr. S, would be doing a transsphenoidal surgery, going up inside Drew's mouth between his top lip and teeth, no visible scars, breaking through to the sphenoid sinus cavity, looking at the tumor through a microtube and suctioning out as much as he could. He doubted he could get it all, but he hoped to get most of it. Since all reports indicated it to be an aggressive tumor, he expected to recommend radiation treatments following surgery, and the radiation would zap the remaining small amount.

"One surgery?" I asked.

"One surgery," he replied. "Chances of needing further operations in this case are about one percent."

Collective sigh of relief. Brain damage, blindness, death—yes, all possible. But somehow it sounded less likely, something that never happened under the steady hand of Dr. S.

Stephen inquired about this man who claimed to be the surgeon.

"Oh yes, I'm glad he came by. That's Dr. T. I've asked him to assist. This particular area of the head is his specialty. No one better. We're lucky to have him." At least he was only assisting, and he was older than he looked.

"Six A.M.," Beth, the nurse told us. "Be here by six if you want to see him before he goes down."

"We'll find you a private room," I promised Drew, stroking his head. "After the surgery we'll work on moving you to the Ritz."

Drew was resigned to a difficult night. He'd told Beth, when she asked, that he wanted the information told to him straight. He'd gotten it straight, even harsh. Sleepless as the night ahead looked, he wanted to be alone. We went home to an all-nighter of our own.

At 6:00 A.M. we arrived in Drew's room and found an empty bed. We'd missed him. They'd picked him up already. No. The three of us clung to the nurses' counter. What could he be feeling, going off all alone, with no last hugs? The staff nurse, with what we found to be a nearly universal compassion from the people in this hospital, called down to the preop room. Yes, they would make an exception. Yes, we could come down and see Drew. Off we zoomed, down elevators, corridors, more corridors, through myriad double doors, to a large warehouse-like room, filling up with people on gurneys, side by side, waiting to be delivered for every possible type of surgery. Most looked half-dead already. Mildly drugged, dressed in pale green cotton wraps, flat on their backs, covered with white sheets, people lay with their eyes closed or focused on nothing in particular. It looked like someone's nightmare in a science fiction scenario.

There at the far end was Drew, waving at us excitedly. Due to low blood pressure, he had not been given sedatives. He was fully alert. He rolled to his side, propped himself up on an elbow, his large blue eyes crinkling at the corners, inviting us toward him. He had had an awful night, bright lights, constant interruptions—blood tests for him, diaper and position changes for his roommate—and a loudspeaker that stopped for rare, too short moments. He was not reticent to tell us he needed us.

We comforted him; he felt safer with us near, this newly formed three-some who seemed to go everywhere together.

A large, serious man came toward us. We thought he would ask us to leave. We'd had our hugs, our soothing reassurances. Instead, with the calm comfort we would see at every turn, he offered us chairs.

The young woman on the next gurney was nineteen. She'd had a seizure out of the blue. There was a tumor in the back of her head. She'd come with her family from upstate New York. I looked at these two beautiful young people, chatting with each other as they might before a class rather than a surgery. What could be causing this?

At 7:00 A.M. they came and took Drew away. "Piece of cake," he told us. "It's you who have to be awake through all this." We each gave him one last kiss. Stephen still remembers this moment with a visceral pang. Stephen has no children of his own and met Drew when Drew was seventeen. Too old for a new father and, if anything, already over-parented, Drew fell into a gray area with Stephen. On the one hand, they became close friends, sharing interests in sports and music. On the other, there was an older–younger man relationship that encompassed advice giving and Stephen's participation in parental decisions. When Drew was spending more time than we thought necessary "exploring his social side," explaining that he didn't feel motivated in school, Stephen calmly but gravely told him, "Getting an education is hard work; motivation has little to do with it. The very notion of motivation is self-indulgent. You just have to get in there and do it—some of it you'll love, some you won't. You do it anyway."

That was the closest Stephen had come to sounding like a real parent. Drew had listened. Mostly they were friends. They actually looked alike, often being mistaken for father and son: two tall, slender men with thick blond hair and open angular faces. As Stephen kissed Drew on that October morning, he felt a new sensation, the gnawing love a parent feels for a child, especially a child in danger.

We left the hospital and went across the street for breakfast. We held reality at bay with croissants and omelettes, fresh strawberries and cream, cup after cup of coffee—foods I never eat and don't even dream about anymore. The date was October 4, 1991, one actual week, one mental decade, since I'd heard the word *tumor* on the phone.

"Between one and two o'clock," the doctor had said. "I'll call down to the family waiting room as soon as it's over," he reassured. The family waiting room. We weren't prepared for the family waiting room, for those stretched-out hours. No way to be prepared. Nothing could make it better. Drew could die, be blinded, be hurt. The week before the schedule was so busy. There had been so many appointments and family and friends to talk to. Drew's college friends had called regularly, sent deluges of artwork, good luck charms, and cards. His dean and advisor called to offer comfort and confide about her own experiences with cancer. Every moment required my full attention. I rarely had the chance to wander from the details at hand.

Now there we were with other, equally stressed families. The room was large, filled with rows of seats facing the volunteer's desk. The volunteer sat cheerfully, sympathetically, answering the phone, calling people over to talk with doctors. That telephone—none has ever been so closely watched, with such anticipation, such dread. I couldn't stand it. We pulled loose chairs into the large entryway and sat around an empty desk in sight of the volunteer but not in her immediate vicinity. What to say, what to do? I'd brought books. My lungs were well enough that I could finally read again, but my brain turned obstinate. We'd talked ourselves out at breakfast. We sat silently surrounded by the endlessness of the next four hours.

Unexpectedly, my brother John arrived. He'd offered to cancel appointments and come. I'd said no; we three were enough. My brother and I weren't very close; he wasn't needed. He's a psychiatrist, familiar with pain. He cleared his schedule anyway and came. He offered comfort and distraction. He told us stories about his closest friend's impending divorce. I was riveted. My friend Nicky, on sabbatical in Vermont, called to check on us from our home. She had come to help.

When she'd first called from Vermont, I'd told her, "You don't need to come. There's nothing for you to do." She came anyway and I'd kept her busy with errands ever since. I sent her off now to prepare nourishing, no-chew foods for Drew postsurgery—plain miso broth in a thermos, mashed millet and sweet squash in a microwave container.

At 1:00 P.M., "There's Drew's doctor," said Stephen.

"No. Are you sure?" I exclaimed. The time was right, but everything else was wrong. He was supposed to call down. Surgeons are tired after surgery; they only come down if the news is bad. Tears started streaming again, silently, down my face. "Drew's dead," I whispered to Stephen. We rushed toward Dr. S, still in his surgery fatigues, small flowers on the fabric.

"Is he all right?" I managed.

"Let's go into the private room over here, and I'll tell you all at the same time."

A blur of faces looked at us pityingly—they still had a chance for success. Dr. S's face was grave. There weren't enough chairs. The wait was maddening. The kindly desk volunteer scurried around finding more. Dr. S's deliberate manner, no doubt a plus in surgery, aggravated me here. Once seated, he told us how successful the surgery had been.

"The tumor is soft tissue. We didn't get it all but between ninety and ninety-nine percent."

Drew was fine. Optic nerve and brain were intact. He wasn't dead, and the chances of further surgery were still around 1 percent. We would never again have to see Dr. E. No open face strip mining needed here. Dr T was finishing up the surgery. Drew would be in intensive care in a couple of hours. My brother John, a doctor, was asking medical questions and getting medical answers. He would be our interpreter. All seemed smooth, in fact celebratory. Then why were we here? Where was the bad news necessitating a family conference? Why not a phone call?

Well, there was something. The tumor was more aggressive than they had expected. Aggressive. That word kept cropping up. What did it mean exactly? Dr. S explained:

"It really means fast-growing. Drew's tumor shows no signs of having spread; it looks self-contained. But it is fast-growing. We will recommend radiation to cover all stray cells. We were surprised, quite frankly, and we're not sure exactly what kind of tumor it is. It's not what we expected. It's not a pituitary tumor. We've brought in a team of pathologists who specialize in rare tissue, and we'll have an answer early, better make it the middle of the week. It's not wise to rush these things. We did see a small mass pushed hard up against the brain. It looks crushed. We didn't remove it because we think it's the pituitary gland."

Think? You *think* it's the pituitary gland, I mumbled to myself. Once again, despite more than a decade of observing the fuzzy edges of medical knowledge, I was amazed at the lack of certainty here. I expected a sure thing. I was getting "we think's" and "maybe's."

We filed out to curious looks and started phoning. Was the news good or bad? We really didn't know. He was alive; he was fine; they got most of it. The news must be good. Everyone was called. Everyone we called had a list of calls to make. The news was good, wasn't it?

As we were packing up to head for intensive care, Dr. T arrived. The terrorist, we had labeled him, he terrified us so much. We looked at him warily, questions flying. Yes, it was over; yes, Drew was fine; he was in recovery now. Dr. T, that self-assured, arrogant man, looked tired. He patiently took all questions, even those with an edge. Andy asked him the question none of us dared ask, the one hard question: "Does aggressive here mean malignant?"

"Yes." Dr. T answered quietly, nearly imperceptibly. He looked so sad, so defeated. We all stood silently.

"We appreciate what you've done for our son," I comforted him, perhaps comforting me. It wasn't his fault it wasn't routine, common, easy to fix.

"Thank you," he said solemnly. Dr. T left us to grapple with the C word, a word we could not yet utter aloud.

So this was the bad news. Drew did not have a benign pituitary tumor. He had a fast-growing, rare form of cancer. Which rare form we wouldn't know for some days. So this is what Dr. S came to tell us. He did tell us. But he did so with such care, so comfortingly, we didn't get it. We didn't get it!

Time passed. We pushed the buzzer for admittance to intensive care. No Drew Todd yet. We were told to wait. We waited. We asked again. "Soon," we were told. We waited. Six P.M. and still no Drew.

"This means there's a problem in recovery," I agonized. "He should have been here hours ago." As I finished this latest lament, a cheerful nurse came up to us. He put his hand on my arm.

"He'll be up soon. There's no problem. They're short-staffed down there, and everyone's come out of surgery at the same time. Your son's fine. I just called down myself to check. They love him down there. He's got everyone laughing. When he comes up, they'll roll him past that window. Give us twenty minutes to get him settled and then ring again."

I adored this nurse in my relief. My fears melted away. I hope he says this to everyone waiting in that room. With such a staff, Drew would be more than cared for; he would be loved. And loved he was. Even the gurney pusher gave my stricken face a thumbs-up sign through the window as I gazed at Drew passing into intensive care, large bandages across his nose, his eyes closed, his face a bluish hue. He looked so vulnerable. Oh, that this could have happened to me instead of him. Don't parents always say that? A Hallmark card sappiness. But it didn't feel sappy; it felt hard, angry, and true. Why him? It was a question I asked repeatedly, a question Drew avoided, finding it defeatist and irrelevant.

Only the parents for the first visit (the unfairness of step-parenting). Andy and I hovered around him. He was hooked up to space age machinery, sipping ginger ale and dozing. He felt no pain. He knew who he was, he recognized us, he could see us, he knew where he was and why. He was still Drew. The inside of his head had been probed and suctioned, but he was still Drew. His roommate, a young woman with long blond hair on one side of her bandaged head, was not so lucky. At intervals she would awaken. Confused by her surroundings, she would rise up, pull out the IVs, the plugs, and assorted attachments, demanding to know where she was. The nurses pulled the curtains between the beds, tried to reassure this distraught young woman, and administered more drugs—perhaps their only alternative but not one geared to reduce confusion.

I focused my attention on Drew. The miseries of those around us kept sending me the message that it could be worse. And it could. Somehow it just didn't feel that way. I concentrated on feeding some miso broth into Drew and gave a nurse the millet mixture. I explained about no hospital food.

"I don't blame you. It's pretty bad," she said. When she smelled the miso soup, she was interested and said, "Macrobiotics. We're seeing more and more of that around here." Drew smiled slightly and was asleep again. I left and Stephen went in. Only two people were allowed in at a time.

At 10:00 P.M. they kicked us out. How could I leave? He needed the security, even when asleep, of our presence. Or was it I who needed his presence? The nurse was sympathetic.

"I'll take good care of him," she reassured me. As I left, she leaned over Drew, stroking his cheek tenderly. "How're you doing, babe?" she cooed. I left partly reassured but (what else?) crying.

In retrospect I see myself as a puddle of tears. Drew recalls it differently. He remembers me as a steady presence, someone he could count on to weather each new blow with him, no matter how shocking, how dreadful. I'm glad for that. For I remember myself as one eternal, if muted, howl.

By noon Drew would be in his new room. I'd badgered admissions repeatedly. I'd requested help from the doctors and nurses. I had been relentless. He had a room in the royalty wing. No roommates, no loudspeaker, a room with a view.

Sally, Drew's stepmother, and Sarah, his eight-year-old sister,* were feeling isolated in California. Sally had known Drew since he was two and a half years old. Sarah had known him all her life. They wanted to be with him. Drew needed them. The crowd was growing. Andy's parents flew up from Washington, D.C., on Friday and sat in their hotel room waiting for news. Sally, Sarah, and a close family friend, Bill, were flying in on Monday. Drew was expected to be in the hospital for a week to ten days.

His room had a small refrigerator. The hospital wing had a microwave. The nurses understood—no hospital food. Just as well; he might have starved. His first hospital meal arrived, unstoppable. His nose was packed and bandaged, so he had no sense of smell or taste. His upper gum was stitched, so he could slowly mash but not chew food. The entree on his lunch tray was roast beef.

My first concoction was ojiya, an energy food to build strength, soft short-grain brown rice simmered and mashed with green onions. At the end I put in one teaspoon of barley miso with a few snippets of kombu, a seaweed rich in iron, calcium, magnesium, and a host of trace minerals. Like yoghurt, miso is full of live cultures. If you boil it or cook it too long, you kill these valuable nutrients. I warmed the brew gently for a couple of minutes, putting it in a wide-mouthed thermos. Drew mostly slept and had no appetite. But he had to eat. In a year he had lost twenty to thirty pounds, and if we didn't feed him, the staff would. Drew figured, in a lucid moment, that this was the time to eat Evelyne's concoctions—while he had no sense of taste or smell. He was making us laugh when he couldn't even smile.

On Sunday the hospital nutritionist stopped by. It was the only day I'd not dressed the part. I was in jeans and a sweatshirt. No one will be around on a Sunday, I thought. I also happened to be giving Drew a foot rub. She looked at me warily.

"Drew's weight, we've got to get it up. What's this special diet you have him on?" the nutritionist asked.

I explained.

"Where are the calories? He needs fat. I am going to put him on a high-calorie milkshake, three times a day."

"No," I yelped. "He's allergic to dairy foods; it's on his chart."

"Okay, we'll make it sugar-based."

*Sarah is the daughter of Drew's father, Andy, and Andy's second wife, Sally. Drew refers to Sarah as his sister rather than the strictly correct half-sister.

"Absolutely not," I said.

This young woman gave me a penetrating look, her whole face a question mark. I could see the tape running through her mind: "Deranged mother, with best of intentions, is starving her child."

"I'll increase the calories. He's not losing weight. He'll gain more easily once he has his appetite back and can chew properly," I assured her.

"I'll give it a few days, but if he loses, I'm ordering supplemental shakes." She left, never to be heard from again. Drew did, however, gain weight without the help of milkshakes.

All that week I woke up early, fixed food in the morning, and went to the hospital. Andy handled breakfast and fed Drew leftovers: soft rice and vegetable mash, carrot ginger soup, split pea stew, mashed pinto beans—healthy baby food. Each day he had some miso soup with fresh vegetables slivered very small, a bit of umeboshi plum paste, a bit of seaweed mixed into one of the soups, and a sweet vegetable drink. Sweet vegetable broth is made by simmering and then straining equal parts of cabbage, onion, sweet winter squash (buttercup, butternut, or acorn), and carrots. Drew drank one-half to one cup of this sweet vegetable broth every day to keep his blood sugar even.

The doctors were, among many things, monitoring Drew's salt levels. The posterior part of his pituitary was weakly functional, but his salts were low. If they dipped too low, it could mean diabetes insipidus, necessitating yet another hormone supplement. He was gradually being put on Synthroid, for thyroid function; prednisone, a hormone for his adrenals; and (later) testosterone. (He also took antiseizure drugs for about one year as a prevention against seizures.) It seemed these supplements would have to be lifelong. The endocrinologist thought his pituitary was permanently nonfunctional, crushed for too long. Dr. S explained that if it wasn't destroyed now, it would be zapped after radiation. To avoid another hormonal supplement we had to build up his salts. Potato chips were suggested for a young man who could barely open his mouth. I had a different idea: Umeboshi plums, a Japanese salted, fermented plum, Drew's single most hated food in the diet, could for now be shoveled in unnoticed, untasted, no guilt. I wasn't torturing my son; I was helping to heal him. His salt levels rose and leveled out, one hormonal drug avoided.

Perhaps keeping me active was one of the appeals of the healing diet. Yes, I was convinced it would help. I had found the studies to suggest it would. I had talked to people who had survived when they weren't supposed to. But there was something else. I was a parent, a mother, and my child was in danger. My role, my passion was to make it go away, make it better. That's what I'd always done. "Tell me where it hurts," I would say. When I fed Drew, he watched me with large, luminous eyes. They seemed to be saying, "I trust you to make this all right." My return look never showed my pain. My eyes said right back to him, "I'm here. It's going to be fine." But once my bedroom door at home was closed, my defeat poured out. I felt powerless. Drew could tell me where it hurt all day, but there was little I could change. One thing I *could* do was cook. I wasn't powerless and passive. Cooking gave me energy and hope, and I could convey this strength to Drew through the food, through my very being. Everything that could be done, drawing on a variety of modalities, was being done. There would be no "we should have's."

We all had our own techniques for creating sanity for ourselves and thus helping Drew. Andy spent all of his time at the hospital, keeping alive their shared interest in sports, announcing new scores, bringing in videos of choice games. Drew, his color returning, sat up between naps to watch these videos, chat with visitors, and make friends with the hospital staff. Sally, Sarah, Bill, and Stephen surrounded Drew with love and were rocks for Andy and me, allowing us to remain steady with each new shock. And the shocks seemed never-ending.

On Sunday, Drew was taken for an MRI. On Monday, Nicky asked if we'd had the results. We hadn't. But what could it show that we didn't already know? Probably 5 percent of the tumor left. So what?

On Tuesday, Dr. T stopped by early. He had been coming in the evenings. He walked in and looked Drew straight in the eye. The MRI had a lot to show.

"We've all taken a look at the MRI. We got most of the tumor, but there's a small mass under the optic chiasm. We're going to have to go in again."

Quiet chaos filtered across each face, except Drew's impassive gaze. "What about the radiation?" we chorused. "Won't that do it?"

"We'll still follow up with radiation, but the mass is too close to the optic nerve—too big a risk of blindness to just use radiation."

A few more statements delivered quickly: He would be making an incision across the top of Drew's head down to his ear, then would probe in from above, moving the brain aside to get to the optic nerve and the remaining tumor. He told us he hadn't decided which side, right or left. *The* brain? He was talking about Drew's brain, moving Drew's brain aside. There was a slim chance that the tumor would drop off the optic nerve and could be irradiated once it was in a less vulnerable part of the head. Dr. T felt that would be most unlikely. He expected to do one more surgery to remove the remaining bulk of the tumor, followed by radiation to clear Drew's head of stray cancer cells.

Who was this annoying man who kept talking as if he were going to be making all of the decisions? Where was our great surgeon? What happened to the one surgery, or the benign pituitary tumor for that matter? Where were all the 1 percent odds? A nurse found us. She explained that Dr. T was known for his lack of bedside manner but was one of the world's great surgeons and we were in good hands. "People come here from every corner of the globe to see him," she said. "He's the best there is for this type of surgery. He just can't talk to people."

He sure couldn't talk to people. But then great surgeons rarely have a reputation as great commiserators. Common wisdom says that doctors can't be too involved because it would be too emotionally draining. I disagree. Nurses do it. They engage empathetically with patients all day, every day. Somehow they have learned to be caring without losing their own emotional or scientific integrity, so it must be possible to maintain an engaged distance if that is your goal. Watching Dr. T, I realized that wasn't his goal. His purpose was to execute brilliant surgery. He was not fascinated by people. He was fascinated by the brain. He worked on people all day, but he was not oriented toward people. Yes, he wanted successful outcomes, and he certainly cared whether people lived or died, whether he found cancer or not, whether the prognosis was positive or negative. But his focus was an intellectual one; he was dazzled by the inner workings of people's heads—people who were anesthetized, sound asleep, out cold. Okay. So that's what we needed him to be the most: a brilliant surgeon, fascinated by his work, who did what he did best in the operating room.

However, when Dr. T came to tell Drew that an unexpected second surgery was necessary, more than two minutes of his time was needed. The same could be said for Dr. S. Dr. S, for all of his soothing manners (so appreciated at times), nonetheless came to tell us Drew had cancer and didn't convey his message. He too, more kindly perhaps, was always on his way out the door. Medical schools are increasing education in communication skills. Few doctors, to date, have had any instruction on how to tell people they have cancer. Medical education is trying to change that. In the meantime perhaps the Dr. T's of the world should do what they do best—great surgery, indulging their enchantment with their organ of choice—and hire great commiserators, people who know the brain (or lung or pancreas) but whose focus is people, colleagues who have time to follow in the wake of the Dr. T's and their unsettling proclamations, explaining, eliciting and answering questions, engaging in that rare event in medical settings—a conversation.

This mythic person was not an option. Given the doctors we were seeing, I had preferred Dr. S. He acted so sure; he looked like he had grandchildren who loved him. But my views were slowly changing. Dr. S stopped by that evening. I observed his reassuring face, his calm gestures, his statistical references, all being talked at us, not with us. We'd needed those that long-distant week ago. Without his careful bedside manner, the stress then would have been unbearable. We were too numb for real dialogue then anyway. He soothed us when it was still possible to do so. Now he irritated me. I didn't want to hear about 1 percent. If you were the 1 percent, it was 100 percent. And Drew seemed to have a pattern of falling into that 1 percent. Comfort didn't work anymore. I wanted someone to look me in the eye and lay it out: "This is what we're dealing with here." My annoyance with Dr. T was decreasing. No, he didn't impart much information, but neither had Dr. S or anyone else for that matter. What he did impart, however, tended to be correct, even if it was an "I don't know." I'd noticed that he didn't bother Drew anymore. They had, in fact, developed a strange, respectful relationship. I'd even seen Dr. T tentatively touch Drew on one of his visits. His manner was unbearable in the first days of this trauma, but now I preferred him. Yes, I wanted more time, more detail, but as for the facts, give them to me cold, and let's have no more high expectations dashed by devastating developments. And please, no more 1 percent odds.

Drew had managed the shocks so far in different ways. All of his responses seemed healthy to me. He had cried in my arms, with his father, and on the phone to Rebecca, who was studying in China. He had drawn strength from his tears and his anger, had looked fate in the face and talked about it. At other times, he went into classic denial. He tried to forget about it. Denial, often gaining a bad rap, can be, at times and in moderation, a natural tranquilizer, a brief respite. But denial works only if you can really take a break. Smiling on the outside while being gnawed on the inside, however, is the negative side of denial. Drew wasn't exactly smiling, but he wasn't talking either. He'd just heard that his head was to be cut open so that a team of surgeons could spend seven to ten hours shuffling his brain around and plucking a malignant growth from his optic nerve, hoping not to blind him, and he was acting like nothing was amiss. But his eyes were scared. We'd respected his responses so far. We did so now, but I was uneasy.

Dr. N, the endocrinologist in charge of his hormonal therapy, came by the day after Dr. T announced the second surgery. She'd just heard the news. She asked us all to leave. (We were quite a mob.) She wanted to talk to Drew alone. She did, for over an hour. A dam burst. For the first time Drew was encouraged by one of his doctors to let go. He told me later that she offered him another side of medical care, one he had rarely seen in his technically oriented medical treatments. Dr. N acknowledged the enormity of Drew's illness and encouraged him to acknowledge it too. She offered him psychological support, support he desperately needed from his doctors—people who had taken over his physical life, his very existence, but shunned his emotional self. Here was a doctor who was a great communicator. Dr. N wasn't a surgeon or a specialist on the brain, but she had another talent; she knew how to listen. Drew took advantage of this rare opportunity and let it all out. The news was too shocking to hold in. He thought it was over, that the worst had been lived through. But the worst hadn't even begun. He'd been told there would be one surgery. He'd expected to be back in school come January. How could he bear this? Would life ever be normal again?

They also talked about medicine. He confided he'd been thinking about medical school. He was a government major, but even before becoming ill, and now especially, he'd become fascinated by medicine, perhaps working with children. She encouraged him. Who could make a better doctor than one who had already seen it all, from the other side? He felt better. He could cope. She came and talked to us. She suggested that we talk with him one at a time, implying, "How can someone play to such an audience?" I loved this woman.

Selfishly, I went in first. He looked better. He repeated the scenario with me and again with Andy, Bill, Sally, and Stephen. Then he felt better. So what—another surgery? He could cope. He felt deeply connected to Dr. N. He was getting sort of used to Dr. T. He could cope.

Repeatedly, Drew was struck down. Each time he carefully made himself strong again. Each time he mourned the news, reached out for or accepted our support, and slowly built himself back up, regaining an upbeat assumption that whatever happened would be all right. He balanced taking an active role in his recovery with accepting the notion that fate was at work here. He juggled responsibility with resignation. He learned to hold on and to let go. He found comfort in his mixture of responses to so much uncertainty and pain. In the next few weeks until the second surgery, he would become increasingly skilled at coping, developing sophisticated strategies for survival—strategies from which we would all learn.

Chapter Four

SURGERY TWO:
HOPING IT WOULDN'T
BLIND HIM

With the arrival of the rest of Drew's family for the surgery, Andy had moved into a nearby hotel. For the first time I was getting to know Drew's sister Sarah. We'd met and visited briefly from time to time, but I really only knew *about* her; I didn't know her well. Now we became friends. I admired her pluck and her ability at the egocentric age of eight to put Drew first, to be quiet in his hospital room, to wait patiently while we ministered to him, often leaving her to amuse herself in strange surroundings for extended periods of time. One afternoon, doctors came and talked with us about the impending second surgery. Sarah sat watching or drawing, saying nothing. We were all too overwhelmed by the discussion of risks and potential pain to look her way. The next day, looking over her shoulder as she wrote a letter to her classmates, I read, "Yesterday doctors came and talked and talked. I've never been so bored in my life." What a kid. What a confusing time this had to be for her. I suggested that Sarah must be suffering ice cream deficiency, and since Drew couldn't have any, she needed lots for both of them. She agreed that this was crucial to his recovery and took off with Stephen in search of her favorite flavor. The week produced a close-knit extended family, bumps and all but close.

Friday, October 11, we had a festive welcome home dinner for Drew and farewell for the Californians. Drew was home from the hospital, his recovery faster than expected.

Everyone had become increasingly interested in Drew's diet. Bill especially felt great after meals I'd fixed. Masao, Evelyne's husband, is a chef. We ordered a takeout vegetarian feast. He made it especially tasty for nonvegetarians and healthy for Drew. We started with a light corn chowder. The main course included greens lightly sautéed in dark sesame oil; brown rice pressure-cooked with fragrant lotus seeds; Arame seaweed and grated carrots in a ginger-tamari sauce, sprinkled with lime zest; Aduki beans in a mold, sweetened with what tasted like mashed sweet squash; and a slivered radish and cabbage pickle. Dessert was a cous-cous cake topped with fresh fruit sauce (not recommended for Drew—still too sweet for the recovery phase). The tastes were balanced with something sweet, sour, bitter, salty, and spicy. The colors were vivid. Masao prepared the food, and Sally arranged the dinner.

Sally is Jewish. She organized a Friday night ritual, a Shabbot. In the Jewish faith Friday night is a family night, a night to pull together, to celebrate the week and each other. It is the woman's night to organize the ceremonies. We sat around the dinner table. Drew, tired but happy to be home, bandages removed, sat at the head of the table. We each took two brilliantly colored fall leaves out of a basket Sally had arranged. With the first we threw off an unwanted part of our lives, returning it to the basket. Second, we celebrated a happiness of the past week. That leaf we kept. Sally lit the candles, we all held hands, those who knew the words sang the songs of Shabbot, and the rest of us hummed along. Then we ate and ate and ate. We felt fine.

I have a friend who does research on how people and families cope with cancer at the Dana-Farber Cancer Institute in Boston. She was surprised that we were all mostly able to pull together in the face of such an intense family drama. Her impression is that serious illness often divides rather than unites people. We did experience tensions. Somehow, however, we achieved a consensus about what was really important (Drew) as opposed to what wasn't (our personal stresses). As a sociologist I pondered influences that might be helping us cope together. Perhaps because we were older, of the same age group, everyone in a stable relationship and in a comfortable career, we could more easily avoid useless competitions. Each set of parents had remarkable friends around and staying with us, who served as unintentional buffers. Most important, Andy, Sally, Stephen, and I shared similar attitudes toward child rearing, medical care, health and illness, and Drew's treatment plans, both conventional and alternative. Together we had enough money to afford often costly explorations that eased the misery—a quiet, comfortable hospital room where nerves were more likely to be soothed than shredded and consultations with such practitioners as the acupuncturist and the macrobiotic nutritionist. Perhaps it was these shared values and resources that gave us the firmest grounding from which to keep our eyes on the main event—Drew's care—as opposed to our individual, occasionally flaring short fuses. Many people with none of these advantages provide loving, supportive care for ill family members, but it is harder and they are more heroic.

My job was on hold. Thanks to my department chair and dean, substitutes were hired for the rest of the semester. I was instructed not to think about work. I was given the luxury of a paid leave in a country where unpaid time off for family illness was still ferociously opposed. I was free to take care of Drew.

The weeks between Drew's return from the hospital after the first surgery (October 11) until his return for the second (November 7) were the most poignant of my life and perhaps his. My friend Robert hates poignant. He prefers movies, literature, people to have some edge. We banter about this; usually I agree with him. In fact it is exactly his edge that I like best about him. But lately the edges in my life had become too sharp. I was settling for poignant.

Once we were three, the house became very still. Stephen shut himself in his study, trying to return to his writing. Drew, pale, thin, and tired, slept long hours. After twenty years of struggling to be a professional woman without a backward glance at the kitchen, I now found myself wanting only to cook. I fixed hearty vegetable stews, morning porridges, and thick bean soups, inventing grain dishes with grains I'd never heard of before. Ethiopians have used teff, the smallest known grain, for centuries. High in protein, iron, and calcium, it has a rich, nutty flavor. Using the dark brown flour to make a pie crust felt like making mud cakes in the backyard.

Another favorite was a creamy millet porridge. One cup of millet, one cup of peeled, chopped sweet butternut or buttercup squash, one-quarter cup of sunflower seeds, a touch of salt, nutmeg and cinnamon, and three cups of water. Simmer for twenty to thirty minutes, then mash. It turns a lovely orangy yellow and is surprisingly sweet, spicy, creamy, and flavorful. On a fall morning it provided a warming, balanced start.

Drew slept and ate and started to feel better than he'd felt in a while. His head seemed clear as energy was seeping back into him. We began to play cards. We'd always been fierce card and game players. We resumed, with no slack given or needed for the ailing. Evening hearts games started with competitive vigor, each of us crowing when triumphant, outrageously aggressive when not. Drew had to get well. Wouldn't anyone let someone really sick win at cards? Could you snicker and gloat at a card player who was dying of cancer? Certainly not. Being beastly at hearts made us all feel better—nearly normal. Perhaps I still had some of that edge Robert had always liked. I wasn't a complete sap, someone who cried in elevators. I could still gloat. I could still laugh uproariously as I captured the queen of spades for my second shot at the moon in one evening.

The doctors were pleased. Drew's quick recovery was unexpectedly smooth. Days were still structured by doctor appointments, blood tests, acupuncture treatments. But frequent, carefully planned meals and relaxation exercises were restful and equally important parts of recovery.

Some researchers claim visualizations can help tumors shrink and ailments heal. Exercises that calm the body and the mind are also great coping strategies. In the hospital Drew had done these twice a day. First Bill and I led him through them; then he did them on his own. Starting with deep breathing, he imagined his body deeply relaxing. Beginning with his feet, he had visualized each part of himself letting go, calming down, nothing to do, nowhere to go, everything at ease. As he relaxed, his breathing slowed, and he visualized his head clear, with healthy cells, the tumor shrinking or dropping off the optic nerve. If the last sticky remnants adhering to the optic nerve would drop and if gravity was on his side, then radiation could be used to zap it, and the second surgery would not be necessary. The healing properties of relaxation exercises are contested by some, but perhaps they would help. One month was a short time to bring about such changes, but these exercises are beneficial on many levels. Regardless of their role in healing, they give a feeling of doing *something*, avoiding that passive patient role, that out-of-control feeling that can lead to hopelessness and depression during illness. It helps to feel actively involved, a team player in your own health. Deep relaxation also feels good. In the midst of such high stress, you get a break, a break that drugs can't give. For with deep relaxation the body feels light and strong, while the mind becomes still but sharp.

In 1986, following a taxi accident that left my back injured and had me flat out for weeks, doctors had offered Valium to calm the muscle spasms and relax me. The drug partly calmed my back but fuzzied my mind. And it was my mind, freed from pain, that I wanted. Lying flat on my back I felt out of control already. To lose a clear head increased this alienation. The result: deeper stress. A physical therapist gave me a relaxation audiotape. I stopped the Valium. Listening to the tape helped decrease the pain while increasing my mental clarity. I hadn't thought much about it since, but once again my own health history was proving invaluable. Was my whole life of pains and gains merely a preview for this main event? It certainly seemed so. Should I reevaluate that taxi accident as a bonus rather than an enraging assault? Well, I wouldn't go that far, but the Chinese characters that define crisis as danger and opportunity or our own "every cloud has a silver lining" seemed applicable here. All of those platitudes I'd relegated to the mindless optimists of the world kept buzzing in my head. In any case we weren't being given choices, so why not grab at the few benefits hidden in the more glaring disasters of these events.

The relaxation, done at bedtime, helped Drew sleep. Night terrors are unavoidable during stress. No matter how often I assured him that if he had a bad night he could wake us for talk and comfort, he never did. Despite being thrown back into the child role, he was, after all, twenty-one. The days of midnight cuddles from nightmares, real or imagined, were over. The deep relaxation exercises, where he visualized himself healed and healthy, helped him avoid the black hole of night. He slept better, so he healed faster.

The doctors were more than pleased; they were surprised. Drew was quickly gaining weight, energy, and color. The supplemental hormones were taking effect, yes, but in addition the visualizations, acupuncture, and diet also had to be helping. I didn't mention all of these "additions" to Drew's doctors. Modern medicine does some things very well. Brain surgery, for example. Doctors adhering to this model do not, however, exhibit the intellectual curiosity for other, complementary approaches to health that I would expect of such brilliant people. I didn't push it. We just rejoiced in the improvements and kept up a steady crusade of our own.

Each moment felt precious, as if it might be our last. To live in the moment and enjoy the present are ideals that sound like good advice. But I now realized I'd seldom lived like that, didn't know how to or even that I wasn't living that way. Now each moment counted. I got a thousand-piece puzzle and set it up in the living room on a card table. Sitting in a sunny window with Drew, both of us poring over that puzzle, listening to bluesy jazz, the only thing that mattered was finding that puzzle piece of green grass. Everything else was muted. "Lila loved puzzles. . . . She always loved the satisfying snap of two pieces going together. It was like knowing something for sure."[1] In Bobbie Ann Mason's elegant novel *Spence and Lila*, Lila is elderly and ill. We, like Lila, toyed with certainty wherever we found it.

Friends and family were also healers. They called, they came, they helped. Locally, our friends were devoted. We didn't experience the withdrawal so many ill people report, especially those with cancer. Drew's friends from school were remarkable. They arrived in twos, threes or fours. They asked Drew right-on-target questions, not avoiding dangerous topics. They were curious. Where had the surgery been? What was he eating? Could they try some? What was acupuncture like? Could they come and watch? The house was full of cards, drawings, and posters from all age groups. A glowing soft-sculpture sunflower hung down one wall in his room, sent by my friends Jane and Shirley, Shirley being a fiber artist. Drew felt loved. How could anyone so loved, so quick to recover, die so young? The tensions were diluted by such devotion.

I found myself having rare opportunities as a parent. I had a second chance, a chance to correct my mistakes, to make up for past shortcomings. How could I have continued watching the movie *Some Like It Hot* on TV when at age six months Drew started to crawl? Why was I ever grumpy with him? Why had I worked on a paper rather than take him to Disneyland that long ago Sunday afternoon? It was only two hours away. How could I so naively have taken for granted his good health, his outliving his parents? Why hadn't I more consciously savored every second? Here was a chance to erase all those wrongs, real or imagined, mostly forgotten, some sharply remembered. Here, indeed, was a second chance.

For Drew's part, gone was the sighed "Oh, Mom" at various suggestions. No longer was the peer group the ever-present focus. His peers, with concentrated exceptions, were away and were busy, attentive but busy. No longer was I busy. We were both a captive audience. Between naps and medical ministrations we went to concerts, dance programs, plays, museums. Stephen joined us when he could, and we became a close threesome seeing the town, the dazzling culture, much of it free, that Boston has to offer. Gone was Drew's skeptical "the ballet?" It had been replaced with the same focused excitement; every moment was important, and fun should be grasped whenever it showed itself, even at dance concerts.

Drew also had unarticulated strategies to keep his spirits up, strategies that we recognize only in retrospect. While living moment to moment, as if life might end any second, he kept one foot firmly planted in the future. There had to be a future, and he always had something he was going to be doing in it.

He spent hours designing a ring for Rebecca. Not an engagement ring, he insisted, perhaps to himself, but a second-year anniversary ring. He examined the ads for ideas, browsed jewelers for the ring he held in his mind's eye. He finally worked with one to make the perfect ring that he could afford. This interest took a lot of time, a lot of fantasizing. After yet another MRI I asked him how he'd held up. MRIs are not painful or frightening tests, but they require stillness in a closed space for forty-five minutes with a loud mechanical noise swirling around your head. For once he'd nearly enjoyed it. He'd planned every detail of the night of the ring—the restaurant, tickets to a show, then home and the ring presentation. He could hardly wait. He did indeed have a future; he had a ring for Rebecca. Rebecca was Drew's lifeline in absence as she had been the year before while with him at Connecticut College. Sometimes two letters arrived in a day. She called; she wrote. Drew clung to the thought of her.

Once he had recovered from his dismay about being in Boston for a second semester, he started making plans. He could have taken a wait-and-see attitude. Would the radiation debilitate him? Should he take it easy? Perhaps a semester off to just relax would be good. Not at all. He looked into taking classes at Suffolk University, where I teach, and signed up for calculus and a film course. No brain damage allowed here. He'd always been intrigued with jazz bass. He talked with a teacher at a local music school and enrolled. Stephen bought him a beret to get him in the mood. He signed up for a future yoga class to help him gently regain his strength after the surgeries were over. My brother John designed a weight program to slowly start building just about every muscle in the body. Drew was to start easy with one-pound soup cans and build up. It was a program that the elderly, the ill, and the weak, as well as the healthy and strong, could benefit from. John put it together in book form. He had been meaning to do so for his clients anyway.[2] This was just the push Drew needed. He read through the exercises and looked forward to being well enough to start. He was cautiously looking ahead. Everything could be canceled if necessary, and he was careful to get necessary rest. He wasn't pushing himself yet. But he wanted a life to look forward to, a life to dream about in that MRI chamber. These were not articulated strategies. Their value emerges only in hindsight. They provided a vision of normality, a security against night terrors. They were plans with a lot of life.

Another future dream fell into his lap between the surgeries. One of his cousins called to offer Drew a Caribbean house for two weeks in March. Her only requirement was that going into the next surgery, Drew visualize aqua waters, silken sands, and a soft trade wind on his skin. He and Rebecca (due to return from China in December) would have a bungalow on the beach perfect for two. Later I came to think that this vision was a main event in what turned out to be a spectacularly smooth and successful surgery.

Stephen and I had taken Drew on a Caribbean vacation, to an island off Puerto Rico, for spring break when he was nineteen. At that time, tearing him away from his college crowd was a feat similar to separating fingers from superglue. Christmas vacation that year had amounted to two dinners together. I wanted more. A trip away from Boston seemed that avenue to more. Drew had always wanted to go to the Caribbean. When I called a travel agent for suggestions, he proposed one of the bigger islands, where we could combine beach and nightlife. I told him he didn't understand. Nightlife would mean crowds, crowds would mean college kids, college kids would mean one with-son dinner, maybe. I wanted an island with no casinos or condos, no free drink on arrival, no time-share plans. We got it. Perhaps if we'd done it when Drew was ten, it would have worked. The trip was fun, but Drew pined for Rebecca, whom he'd just started seeing, and for the nightlife I'd avoided. Here was his second chance. A perfect vacation.

We still hadn't mentioned cancer. Drew hadn't asked, and we hadn't offered. The lab results were uncertain. All that uncertainty again. My friend Archie Brodsky co-authored a book on the need for medical professionals and the public to accept uncertainty in health and illness.[3] Uncertainty is always present. To continue to pretend otherwise under layers of medical mystifications is detrimental to making the best possible choices in health and thus in life. In my own research I'd seen doctors give people a diagnosis and prescription with absolute certainty, later telling me how unclear they were about the problem, its cause, and thus its cure. Although we all want a sure thing, I agreed with Archie. Certainty is rarely available, and to pretend it is can be harmful to people and to health care. I'd talked about this in classes. With great certainty I'd lectured on the need to acknowledge uncertainty.

So it was with at least some irony that I assailed these new unknowns in my life. Hadn't the best neuropathologists taken a week longer than expected to look at this tumor? Of the three possible categories, why couldn't they settle on one? Yes, it was malignant, we'd been told that after the surgery. But how malignant? Which of the two possible tumor types—chordoma or chondrosarcoma—was it? Would it respond to the radiation or not? The answers, when they finally came, were vague, uncertain. Dr. T called. Stephen, Drew, and I were on the phone. He sounded grave. Granted he was not a man given to light banter, but occasionally he sounded more serious, sadder than usual. It always meant trouble. Dr. T explained the pathologists thought the tumor to be a chondrosarcoma. They wouldn't commit to a definite category but they were calling it a grade 2.

Chondrosarcomas are classified as a form of bone cancer despite being soft tissue that actually grows out of the bone and cartilage. Such cancers are usually located in the pelvis, upper leg, or shoulder and most commonly occur in people over age forty. Only 3.8 percent of this type of cancer appears in people Drew's age and younger. Bone cancers in general are rare; chondrosarcomas are rarer. Still more unusual is to find them in the young, especially in the sphenoid sinus area of the head. The grade of the tumor can be 1, 2, or 3, from least to most serious. Most tumors of this type fall into the grade 1 or 2 areas. Grade 3 generally means malignant, metastasized (spread), unresponsive to radiation, and terminal.[4] Studies on how to treat chondrosarcomas in the head are rare, as rare as the tumors themselves: "The relatively infrequent occurrence of these tumors plus their diverse histology and diverse presentations have made it difficult for any one institution to have enough patients to directly compare, in a randomized prospective fashion, one treatment with another to determine the optimal primary therapy."[5] But studies of successful treatments are in progress for grades 1 and 2 tumors—surgery and proton beam radiation—based on five-year survival rates.

Dr. T explained that Drew's radiation would proceed anyway, despite the uncertainties after recovery from the next surgery; the tumor did not seem to have metastasized. I wanted to ask the scary questions: Was there a chance it was a grade 3? What was the "anyway" in the radiation decision? Anyway, it might not work? On and on. Dr. T was a man of few words; I could have talked all night. But I was silent. Drew was on the phone. He wasn't asking. He had to be the one to open those doors. If he had been five years old, I could have talked with the doctor alone and presented selective information. But Dr. T was talking with Drew. Drew was his patient, and I was lost in the background noise.

Drew was optimistic. He'd heard it differently. I was glad I hadn't inserted my own troubled mind into his. He hadn't heard the unknowns, the "anyway," the sad sounds in Dr. T's voice. He'd heard "radiation," "not metastasized," translated into fixable. Drew got certainty. I didn't, but I was grateful he had. His indomitable spirit was soaring, and perhaps all that jabber about positive thinking would prevail.

I'm not against positive thinking, but it's not enough. The emphasis on patient responsibility—found in questions such as "What are you doing to make yourself sick?"—blames the victim, burdening the already ill person with added stigma, guilt, and stress. There is a fine line between encouraging people to take responsibility for helping themselves and blaming them when sickness occurs.

Mind-body research in this area shows great promise but can also fall into a "blame the patient" trap. Woven throughout current articles and books is a call to turn passive patients into active persons with some control over their own health—a call to be applauded. But often, before you can arrive at these comforting methods and the data that support them, you first have to wade through statements like "in the coming decade, the most important determinants of health and longevity will be the personal choices made by each individual," and these choices can "offer an individual great insight into why he or she 'needs' a disease or symptom."[6] Or the following statement (made uncritically) in an article in *Ms.* magazine on useful nonsurgical remedies for women with fibroids: "[Dr.] Ballantine . . . prefers to begin treatment by asking, 'What is a woman doing psychologically to tie herself up in knots and become excessively fibrous?'"[7]

Such assumptions of individual control and blame bring to mind Louise Lasser in an episode of that mid-1970s parody of all that is wrong with the modern age, "Mary Hartman, Mary Hartman." Mary is eagerly holding onto a firmly entrenched table while being advised by her est coach that if she just tries harder, if she just believes, she can continue to hold onto the table and walk across the room at the same time. When she cannot pull this off, she's told she's not trying hard enough.

These notions of individual culpability increasingly permeate both alternative and conventional medicines. Statements regarding personal choices and illnesses are made in a way that makes them seem perfectly reasonable. But they are not. Yes, we can make healthy and unhealthy choices. Certainly, one of the purposes of this book is to show just how crucial one's actions are in coping with and recovering from illness. But there are larger issues as well when considering why so many Americans suffer from rising rates of cancer and chronic disease. The air we breathe, the chemical feasts in our environment and food supply, and for many the economic arrangements—poverty, lack of access to adequate health care, and so on—also crucially affect personal and societal health. We live in a society that sells us bad health and then blames us for not taking care of ourselves. If attitudes and behaviors are related to health, enhancement of these attitudes and behaviors will have to come from many directions, both societal and individual.

Analyses that incorrectly assume that we can individually cure all that ails us by just doing and thinking the right things can cause great damage. If the prevailing view is just to change ourselves, we risk losing sight of the serious need for social, environmental, political, and economic reform. Why clean up toxic waste if loving oneself is all that's needed?

Zealous emphasis on mind over matter, positive thinking over reasonable possibilities, is a fallacy seen in many areas of modern American life. The emphasis on individual life-style in health pulls on the idea (indeed, the hope, one I understand all too well) that we can dominate our destinies, striking a responsive chord that goes to the very heart of Western values.

It is particularly unfortunate when an overemphasis on the "you can do anything if you try hard enough" attitude slips into health care, however, for if the mind is as important to health as at least some current writers believe, surely such blame-the-victim ideologies set people up to feel like failures when, despite a complete makeover and positive attitude, the cancer is still there. This can only introduce guilt, increase stress, and thus risk worsening health. Guilt among mass murderers or child abusers, so rarely present, is appropriate. Guilt among people with cancer, all too frequent, is not.

But all of these ideological and political debates were unknown to

Drew. He wasn't consciously working at positive thinking, and I don't think it ever occurred to him to connect self-love or lack of it to his illness. He had always been a sunbeam, and his basic personality, amid sporadic emotional distress, won the day. Perhaps this is too simple or remembered through a falsely rose-colored lens. It was such a complicated time. Each moment was a struggle manifested in tears, long talks, many hugs, raw nerves filled with edgy moments. There were lots of edgy moments. For example, the time Stephen and I erupted into an angry fight about affirmative action—an important issue but not the real focus of our rage. After twenty minutes we dissolved in tears. Our anger was at fate, our rage at cancer.

In his father's household Drew had learned to explore and express his feelings from an early age. Too much and too well, I had sometimes thought. Sally in particular had encouraged him to explore the inner life, not to hold back, to let it all out, to know what he was feeling and to act on it. Coming from a critical, sociological framework that permeated my life as well as my work, I had always encouraged Drew to look outward, assessing and questioning the world around him. When he was quite young, I would analyze children's movies for him, how negatively people of color were portrayed or how unequally girls and boys often were treated. This resulted, not surprisingly, in his refusing for a time to go to movies with me. But some of this influence had stuck. As he got older, he loved debating everything from film to politics. Rebecca, at one of her first dinners with us, laughed after a heated debate on current politics and said, "Now I know where Drew gets his political fire from, his feistiness over things I used to rarely think about."

Somehow these influences were being played out, meshed together, to deal with tough times. He wanted to know everything. "Why radiation over chemotherapy? What's the difference? Will there be other people my age there? Are there support groups for what I have?" He questioned each decision and expressed his feelings—sometimes rage, sometimes sadness, other times enjoyment of the moment, always fear. "Sometimes I think about dying, and it scares the hell out of me. But I try to just let it go. I can't control that. If I die, I die. I have to do everything I can to live and leave dying up to fate—that's fate's problem, not mine."

What I hadn't known about Drew was how capable he would be under pressure. He was using intricate coping strategies that allowed information to seep into him in doses he could assimilate. He heard what we heard, but he heard it in a way he could tolerate. The terrors were there, but he wasn't going to let them dominate. He would handle them on his own terms. He would face them incrementally. We didn't push it. When he was ready to talk about cancer, we would know it. We got off the phone with Dr. T and played a ferocious game of cribbage. For once I didn't mind losing.

Support continued to pour in from friends and family. People who prayed were praying, were in fact having their whole congregations pray. Stephen's friend John from graduate school days, our most seriously religious friend, even did a novena. He wore a small pebble in his shoe to remind him to pray for Drew throughout the day. Friends had gatherings where they talked about Drew and hoped for his recovery. Friends at Connecticut College held a meeting in the College House, where they focused on his health and healing. Others concentrated, visualized, hoped that last bit of tumor would shrink and/or drop down into some safe cavity where the radiation could prevail. What a strange road to find myself on—looking to, indeed yearning for radiation, that powerful, threatening force that kills as well as cures, as the answer for all our hopes, hopes that the last smidgen of tumor would drop and radiation alone would be needed.

It was not to be. Surgery was scheduled for Friday, November 8. Monday, November 4, Drew had another MRI. We took the new pictures to Dr. T's office. I explained that we needed to hear immediately so that Drew's California family could finalize their plans. Dr. T's unfailingly kind secretary looked me in the eye, saying, "I understand." "Yes," I admitted sheepishly, "I too need to know as soon as possible." Dr. T was in surgery, but he would call when done. He did.

I'd told Stephen one night that although I knew I needed to be prepared for the worst, I wasn't and wasn't able to be. I warned him that if they had to cut open Drew's head, I didn't know how I could bear it. Since I had to be strong to help Drew, the real sufferer here, Stephen needed to understand my terror to help me help Drew. I had to warn Stephen that while all medical knowledge, logic, and intellect said the tumor would still be there, I, in my deepest places, believed it would not. I wanted to be prepared, but I didn't know how.

"Yes," Dr. T said, the tumor was still there, as he expected it would be, so surgery was set for Friday; check-in time, 1:00 P.M. Thursday, business as usual. I was devastated. Stephen was his usual rock of support, and I was able to help a resigned Drew get ready. At least this time we knew more; we had more time. Despite my certainty that this surgery would be unnecessary, we were prepared.

So the tumor hadn't shrunk, but it hadn't grown either. This was good news. Enough time had lapsed for some growth from such an aggressive cancer. We grabbed at what we could for comfort and hope.

This surgery was to be longer, more fraught with risk, more dramatic. Seven to ten hours. Dr. T would spend hours plucking sticky tissue from Drew's optic nerve, hoping it wouldn't blind him. Great. Hoping it wouldn't blind him.

Despite the increased dangers, we were less terrified or perhaps more numb. We weren't being carried along by the high trauma, the newness, of life-threatening illness. Life-threatening illness, rather, was now the norm, something we never got used to but that was woven into the fabric of our daily life. In fact, the second surgery is less clear in my memory, less etched detail by detail, than either the first surgery or the time between.

I remember one night a week before the second surgery when Drew, Stephen, and I went to an exhibit of the Cone sisters' collection at the Museum of Fine Arts in Boston. The paintings were mainly Matisse: bright colors, women with a strong eye watching you looking at them. I remember the soft peach and mauve walls, the gray carpet; I remember exactly what we had for dinner, plotting how to get the recipe for the salmon exquisitely placed on a bed of perfectly spiced lentils and colorful vegetables. How contented the three of us felt at being out on the town, looking like healthy people without a care in the world. In fact, a friend we ran into remembers Drew aglow, laughing, looking like a Matisse painting himself.

I have no such clear memories of the second surgery itself. This time everything was preplanned. Andy, Sally, Sarah, and Bill stayed at a hotel near the hospital. This time we avoided the family waiting room. During the morning of the surgery we went to the hotel. I dozed, others worked out in the gym, and we ate a lot of ridiculous things—I can't remember what. Dr. T had been kinder the night before: he had touched Drew's foot with affection, it seemed to me. That long, lean foot that was so much the foot of a man when in large, bulky athletic shoes now looked vulnerably slender under the sturdy, dark-haired hand of Dr. T. The hospital staff was kind; the room was lovely. Somehow over the past weeks I had stopped crying. No one seemed to be sleeping much, but otherwise we must have glided along, even though I don't remember it all. Drew doesn't either. He felt resigned to whatever would happen. He daydreamed about Caribbean breezes, hoping he would be able to see the aqua water.

The surgery started at 7:00 A.M. and was due to be over between 4:00 and 6:00 P.M. Around 1:00 P.M. we returned to the hospital. This part is clearer. My brother John arrived with distractions. He had no new friends' divorces with which to entertain me, but he brought a portable CD player and a variety of discs. Stephen read, I listened to music, John watched, everyone else went for food. A little after two the volunteer came over and said the doctor had called down and left a message. This I remember clearly. "It's too early," my stomach muscles screamed.

"They've given up," I moaned.

"No," she said. Drew was in recovery, but where they had put him seemed strange to her. "Maybe they plan to keep him overnight," she offered, a statement that afforded me no comfort. "The doctor will call back shortly."

John went in search of everyone while Stephen and I hovered by the desk. The doctor called again. I took the phone in the private consultation room, and Stephen was on the desk phone. At least the doctor was calling, not coming. Would they tell me bad news on the phone? Oh please, no.

"We're all done," Dr. T fairly sang. "We got it all. Drew's fine. It was a very successful surgery; he's in recovery now, and he'll be up in intensive care in a couple of hours. Everything went smoothly." Dr. T sounded excited, relieved; the surgery must have been even riskier than we had known. Despite all, it went well, it went quickly. Dr. T had the satisfaction of saving a life or preventing blindness; we had the euphoria of an intact Drew. This I remember distinctly.

I ran out of the private room, sobbing loudly—no more silent tears streaming down my face. Stephen and I yelped and embraced. Out of the corner of my eye I saw John with everyone else across the room looking panicked. After all it was only 2:30, and I was sobbing and holding onto Stephen. I yelled across the room, "It's great. He's fine. It's over." We all hugged and yelled, watched with momentary envy and sympathy by the waiting crowd. No doubt this is a room used to a variety of outbursts, but I'd never envisioned myself sobbing, yelling, jumping up and down in a room full of strangers, regardless of the circumstances.

The rest is a haze with a few more of these sharp memories. This time the top of Drew's head was bandaged, his beautiful face extremely white but otherwise unscathed. Dr. T, that ever-somber presence, came to see Drew that night, walking jauntily down the hall, hands in pockets, whistling. He was the friendliest he had ever been. Drew was not only a likable guy and an interesting patient (medically speaking), he was a success story. We sure loved Dr. T that night. We were all happy that it was a success story.

Despite our euphoria, Drew, for the first time, was more remote. In the hospital he wanted more quiet. He asked his father to talk more softly. Grumpy is too strong; detached is more like it. He seemed to have hit that existential realization that at some level he was alone in this. We could all love him and care for him, but we didn't have a tumor in our heads, we wouldn't be needing two months of proton beam radiation at levels higher than it was previously thought the human body could tolerate and perhaps were too high; the studies were optimistic but went back only five years. We weren't the ones who were going to miss graduation with our friends; we weren't at risk. No, at a deep, untouchable place, he was indeed alone. He explored this new consciousness quietly. He kept to himself. No new friends among the nurses, no smiles, no tears, no interests, just sleep and the need for quiet. We did our best, but I am of the school of "Tell me where it hurts." I already had faced the agony of not being able to make it better, but that didn't prevent attempts, at times frantic ones, to do so. I had to sit on myself, as did everyone else, to let it ride, to allow Drew to come to terms with something none of us could really understand, to be there when he needed us and to go away when he didn't.

It was into these uncertain waters that my friend Cathy arrived from California. She and Drew were old friends, having met in 1975, when Drew was five. He would paddle along after us, often annoyed that we talked so much with each other instead of to him. But Cathy is one of those rare adults who treat children as just one of the gang. I remember a chilly afternoon in 1978 when she plotted with Drew to burn all of her thick phone books in the fireplace after the wood ran out. Page by page, they built brief, brilliant flames, probably putting us all at risk of paper fires and toxic fumes but obliviously so. Drew, of course, loved her. Today Cathy's a filmmaker. Her award-winning 1991 documentary *Maria's Story*, about the struggles in El Salvador seen through the eyes of one woman, was on PBS and making the rounds of local movie houses. Drew, before realizing he was ill, had arranged for her to come to

Connecticut College in November, show the film, give a talk, and run a seminar on filmmaking. As it happened, he was in the hospital for this event. Cathy went anyway.

Cathy had called and wanted to stay in Boston before and after the presentation for as long as I needed her. With what was becoming my usual lack of self-knowledge in these matters, I told her I wasn't certain about houseguests now and there wasn't anything she could really do. She had a suggestion: two nights in Boston, two in Connecticut, three in Boston; and if staying with us was hard, she'd move to a hotel and sightsee. Okay. She came and instantly saw that Drew didn't want to talk about surgery. They talked about film. After her trip to Connecticut, she entertained him with every detail of her visit. She'd met and liked all of his friends. They gossiped, they laughed, they discussed Latin American politics. Drew slept. His friends called: they liked Cathy. They loved *Maria's Story*. His visit to the bottomless pit, that hotel anomie, if not over, was at bay. Cathy cooked and commiserated. When Saturday came, I lamented, "Why are you going home so soon?"

Chapter Five

AMERICANS CAN'T
EAT THIS WAY

How is it that you're always so well, so lively?" the wife of one of Drew's fellow radiation patients asked him one morning before treatment, about four weeks into his radiation.

Radiation at the cyclotron lab and at the hospital was not unlike William Hurt's experiences in the movie *Doctor*: people sitting around waiting their turn, chatting about their cancers, their side effects. On the first day of Drew's radiation in December 1991, he, Rebecca, and I had set off wary of yet another unknown, prepared to be unprepared. A large woman in her thirties sat with one leg tucked under her, her elbow resting on a white bed pillow, her face blotched with dark butterfly-shaped marks spreading from one cheek, across the bridge of her nose, to the other cheek. She looked at us sympathetically,

"Is this your first time?" she asked all of us, perhaps not sure who the patient was. (Drew's hair was shaped in a bowl cut, reminiscent of his childhood, that left the scar from his second surgery undetectable). Drew answered yes as he was called back for his first treatment by a warm young man intent on reassurance.

"We'll have him back here in about 45 minutes," the young man explained. "Help yourselves to coffee and cake."

I asked the woman how she was and what she was being treated for. I had learned from Drew that he felt uncomfortable with the avoidance small talk we have all resorted to when confronted with frightening circumstances. He found direct questions easier. This woman seemed to also.

"I'm not doing so great," she replied and went on to describe the tumor in the side of her head that her doctors had only partially removed.

"How long have you been receiving radiation?" Rebecca asked.

"Six weeks, and I don't know if it's the cancer or the radiation that's killing me. The first three weeks were okay, and then everything fell apart."

"What happened?" I asked, both wanting and not wanting to know.

"Well, there's the nausea. It comes and it goes. But worse is the metal taste in my mouth all the time. It makes everything taste the same, and I can hardly stand it. Lately I've been getting headaches, and about a week ago my face started changing colors. I'm so tired all the time and can't do nothing, so I guess I'm not doing too good."

Rebecca and I sat appropriately subdued by her testimony and appearance. Was this going to happen to Drew? Did he have only three weeks before he would fall apart too? So much to fear.

Everyone in this clinic was having proton beam radiation, a finely focused, high-intensity beam. There are three such centers in the country, two in California and one in Boston. General radiation starts at peak strong, damaging tissue as it goes, finally hitting the designated area with its weakest shot. Proton beam radiation does the opposite. It starts weak, gathering momentum, saving its strongest jolt for the target. In other words, the impact is where it needs to be. It is believed to be more precise and focused, with fewer adverse side effects.

Proton beam radiation requires extensive preparation, using MRIs, CAT scans, the making of a head mold for each patient, and other steps. Researchers in the field describe it as follows:

Proton beam treatment techniques provide a powerful approach to improving dose distribution (decrease treatment volume towards target volume) and hence increasing dose to target with resultant higher tumor control rates and lesser morbidity. To achieve these dose distributions in patients requires use of modern imaging techniques, rigid immobilization systems, confirmation of target position vis-a-vis the proton beam at each treatment session, treatment planning which features beam's eye view, displays of uncertainty, dose at each anatomic point, boli based on accurate assessment of density along each pixel, etc.[1]

Early studies had shown radiation to be ineffective on chondrosarcomas (Drew's type of cancer). More recent applications, using higher levels of radiation than previously thought possible (66.6 gray over 37 visits in Drew's case), showed promising results. "The results of high dose proton treatment of chordomas and low grade chondrosarcomas of the base of the skull is particularly promising: an actuarial 5-year local control of 78% has been obtained in 50 patients followed for a minimum of 22 months."[2] Only more years and more patients would tell whether the good results were sustainable, whether the human body could indeed tolerate such high dosages of radiation.

What had seemed so mysterious became familiar once surrounded by a culture of cancer. Most of the people Drew met had their share of stories. Side effects, perhaps milder than from standard radiation, still ranged from fatigue and nausea to blinding headaches, lack of appetite, metallic tastes, hair loss, blotchy skin, and so forth. Except for minor hair loss and occasional fatigue, Drew experienced none of these.

"Seaweed," Drew answered the inquiring wife offhandedly.

She wrote down his instructions and looked eager. Her husband, ignoring the conversation, studied his magazine a bit too intently. He looked as though he was thinking, "Not likely." Diet was, once again, important for Drew. Granted he was young and previously strong, but so were others, coming and going, discussing their reactions, feeling lousy. I wanted to help them, but my remedies were exotic, the doctors knew nothing about them, and the patients felt too ill to start experimenting.

The radiotherapist, Dr. R, had shrugged when we asked about foods.

"Eat a balanced diet. Keep the weight up. That's all."

But what is a balanced diet today? When I was in grade school in the 1950s, the grid showing the four food groups (fruits and vegetables, proteins, dairy, grains) included lots of cows—cows for meat, cows for milk. We were instructed to flood ourselves with protein and fat. Few of us realized then that the four food groups were not written in stone from some wise source but rather were derived by the dairy industry to boost their bottom line.[3] Even osteoporosis, where dairy is pushed as the major prevention, is seen by some as not so much a calcium deficit as a protein overdose.[4] The growing trend among researchers, filtering down through the popular press, is that if you eat this original version of a "balanced diet," you are likely to live sicker and die younger. Your chances of contributing to the heart and cancer statistics rise. Studies of young Americans today, for example, show that all children reviewed had worrisome fatty deposits in their coronary arteries, leading researchers to conclude that this is a universal problem among American children and teenagers. Cause: childhood diets rich in fast-food fats.[5]

As early as 1979, the U.S. Surgeon General's report on "health promotion and disease prevention," called for less fat, sugar, salt, and processed foods and more fresh vegetables, fish, whole grains, and legumes.[6] The surgeon general reported that American vegetarians and people in other countries who ate variations on this recommended diet had less heart disease. The American Heart Association agreed.

This report came in the wake of a Senate Select Committee on Nutrition and Human Needs publication, *Dietary Goals for the United States*, published in 1977. This report suggested greatly reducing fats, sugars, and salts and increasing complex carbohydrates.

The diet of the American people has become increasingly rich—rich in meat, other sources of saturated fat and cholesterol, and in sugar. . . . The risks associated with eating this diet are demonstrably large. The question to be asked, therefore, is not why should we change our diet but why not? . . . . [H]eart disease, cancer, diabetes and hypertension are the diseases that kill us. They are epidemic in our population. We cannot afford to temporize. We have an obligation to inform the public of the current state of knowledge and to assist the public in making the correct food choices. To do less is to avoid our responsibility.[7]

The response to these suggestions was largely negative. The Dairy Council, as well as the egg, meat, salt, and sugar industries, all predictably dismissed such goals. Somewhat less predictably the American Medical Association also dissented: "there is potential for harmful effects from a radical long-term dietary change as would occur through adoption of the proposed national goals."[8]

Despite such resistance, investigations into the relationship between what we eat and our health continued. The National Academy of Sciences issued a landmark report in 1982, *Diet, Nutrition and Cancer*.[9] For some years I have lectured from this report to medical sociology classes. Students are routinely interested and surprised at the information. Diet and heart disease, yes. But cancer? Aside from increasing beta carotene (found in vegetables such as broccoli and carrots), is there a connection? Yes, says this body of scientists, whose report until recently was largely ignored. In a 472-page document, their salient point is that most modern cancers are linked to modern diet—an abundance of animal foods (dairy and meat products) and thus saturated fats, enormous sugar consumption, and perhaps worst, the myriad chemical additives that we know so little about and that are so pervasive in our food supply. Different foods are linked to different cancers: high fats to breast and colon cancer, high use of smoked or salt-cured foods to stomach and esophagus cancers, and red meat to prostate cancer. They also took a skeptical look at our food additives and the lack of adequate testing to assess effects on the body.

Indeed, other cultures eating a more "primitive" diet seem to fare better when it comes to cancers and heart disease. The Hunzas, by now famous, living in a remote corner of India in the Himalayan mountains, are generally used as an example. These people eat whole grain foods, lots of leafy green vegetables, beans and nuts, apricots, and occasional animal foods such as yogurt. The standard Indian diet, full of spices, sugars, refined rice, lots of fats, and black teas, is not eaten there. The Hunza are the only people I've read about who are truly healthy: no chronic or infectious diseases; long, active lives; looking and acting much younger than their age (some over one hundred years old and still working in the fields). Granted, working in the fields at age one hundred may not appeal to some of us, but being healthy enough to do so does. In 1922 the *Journal of the American Medical Association* published the first reports about these extraordinary people.

In 1927 an English physician in India, Robert McCarrison, intrigued by such a healthy population, conducted a study on rats. He gave one group the standard Indian diet. These unfortunate rats developed heart disease, cancers, cysts, and all of the ills that show up in the modern age. The Hunza-diet rats thrived, remaining as healthy as the Hunza themselves.[10] Following these rather dramatic findings, the Hunza people received a bit more attention and then were largely forgotten by the research world until the recent National Academy of Sciences report mentioned above.

Closer to home, the Tarahumaras, in north central Mexico, are considered the healthiest North Americans. "The Tarahumara Indians of Mexico attract special medical attention because of their remarkable physical endurance and their diet which contains very little food from animal sources."[11] The average Tarahumara's diet consists of corn, beans, squashes, vegetables. They occasionally eat meat and eggs. Their work (farming) and sport (kickball) are highly active. Modernity has passed them by, like the Hunzas, in way of life and disease.

Even where modernity is firmly entrenched, with all that it has to offer (which is considerable) and all that it does to harm, diet makes a difference. Rates of degenerative diseases in Great Britain decreased during World War II; cancers declined. Sugar, meat, and fatty foods were scarce, whereas vegetable and grain consumption increased. Following the war, with the end of rationing and a return to a more "affluent" diet, these disease rates slowly climbed back to prewar levels.[12] No one would suggest that war is the road to good health, but useful information turns up in unlikely places. Similar results were found in a more recent study in Cambridge, Massachusetts, during a time of relative peace, at least in North America. Twenty-one people on macrobiotic diets had minimal cholesterol levels. When 250 grams of beef were added daily to their diets, their total plasma cholesterol levels rose by 19 percent, and their systolic blood pressure increased significantly. Once returned to their normal diet—vegetarian, low in fat—their bodies stabilized, cholesterol and blood pressure returning to previous levels.[13]

After I started teaching about connections between nutrition and health, I discovered that the politics involved were equally interesting. Despite the 1982 National Academy of Sciences report, authored by prestigious scientists—no New Age, alternative gurus here—the American Cancer Society continued to deny links between cancer and diet. Their recipe brochure included items such as a cheesy hamburger casserole. The emphasis was lots of fat to offset weight loss in cancer patients and lots of protein for energy. We have moved forward. Recently, in a dormitory at Connecticut College there was a poster covered with vegetables—carrots, leafy greens, broccoli, and so forth. The heading: Prevent Cancer. The sponsor: the American Cancer Society. But we still have a long way to go. The emphasis in the media and medicine is on individual change. If each of us lives better, we won't get sick. Dr. Samuel Broder, director of the National Cancer Institute, is billed as the "government's top cancer doctor." To decrease our high cancer rates, he advises continued cancer research and changes in life-style. "And people should stop smoking, eat and exercise better and take more occupational precautions if they are exposed to known carcinogens. Individuals have to take responsibility for their own health."[14] Perhaps. But our society still pushes us toward all that ails us. Educational materials for grade schools are still "the four food groups," albeit revised. Restaurants, for the most part, offer standard American fare. Advertising gives us contradictory messages to keep fit (join a health club, buy athletic clothes), slim down (join a diet center), and eat sweet and fatty foods (fast foods on every corner). Grocery stores sell mostly processed foods, animal products, and sweets. The large produce sections present fruits and vegetables grown in ever weaker, chemicalized soils and sprayed with poisons that increasingly don't seem to bother the bugs (they have quick genetic adaptability) but may be killing us. Many people work too hard to have time to cook. They rely on fast foods and frozen dinners, just the foods we're being told to avoid.

When Dean Ornish, best-selling author of a healthy heart diet,[15] is challenged by his fellow doctors, saying that Americans can't eat his way (similar to macrobiotics), he answers, "Ask them. Give people the choice." He's right; he's talking about life and death. Under these conditions many people might choose life. What Dr. Ornish doesn't argue for, however, is a way to make it easier for us, the public, to choose to be healthy. His emphasis on individual responsibility for illness ignores social responsibility. Our environment is hardly healthy or amenable to individual change. Even if we want to eat better, it isn't easy. How do we eat better when the food is laced with carcinogens and organic foods are scarce and expensive? How do we take "occupational precautions" against pervasive toxic chemicals built into buildings and carpets, whether at home or at work?

Broder, Ornish, and the rest of us need to be calling for more sweeping changes—changes in food production, the building industry, and so forth. What we need is industrial and societal change to make individual change possible. Individual responsibility requires corporate and government responsibility. It would help, for example, if carpeting chemicals were better regulated so that people could enter new buildings and not risk unhealthy exposures. It would be a lot easier when emerging from the subway if, along with the doughnut shop and hamburger/sub joint, we could find a place to buy a bowl of pasta stir-fried in a little olive oil, with fresh mixed vegetables and sesame seeds or a cup of miso soup. Miso soup may be an acquired taste, but knowing that scientists have discovered in fermented soybeans (miso) the compound (genistein) that inhibits capillary—and thus tumor—growth could make it more quickly delicious; the deep-fried doughnut more odious. After all, wouldn't it be great if we were given the choice? Our health needs to be viewed as equally dependent on cultural choices and personal habits. In fact, personal habits are themselves found in the larger context of societal choices.

As a society, we lose at both ends of the statistical spectrum. At one end we are an affluent society with rich foods, fast foods, and little exercise, contributing to high rates of industrial, modern disease. At the other end of our spectrum we have poverty, with not enough of any food or health care, resulting in appalling illness and death rates in areas associated with poverty, such as infant mortality.

Thus, when Dr. R suggested a balanced diet, what did he mean? "Eat what you want, what you feel like" was the response. After surveying the evidence, Drew didn't exactly eat what his stomach felt like— pizza and Boston cream pie still had their attractions—but he did eat what he wanted, or at least what his intellect wanted him to eat to get well once exposed to information on diet and cancer.

In her book about healing herself from cancer with diet, Elaine Nussbaum reports: "I had spent so much time in the hospital. Countless doctors had asked me a myriad of questions about my past. No one had ever asked me what I was eating."[16] No one asked Drew either. Lack of interest, not resistance, seemed to be the response if any of us asked probing questions or offered information. If Drew wanted to eat seaweed and he thought it made him feel better, "fine," was the attitude. We encountered no curiosity about research and scientific studies (usually a lure in medical circles) that document the positive effects of these antidotes, many from Japan.

No people in the world have had more dealings with radiation than the Japanese. Since the World War II bombs on Nagasaki and Hiroshima, researchers in Japan have done extensive studies of effects of radiation on the body, whether from bombs or cancer treatments, and of how to mitigate those effects.

Dr. Tatsuichiro Akizuki, a physician in charge of the department of internal medicine at a Nagasaki hospital, successfully treated survivors of the nuclear bomb in his hospital who were suffering from radiation fallout sickness. Dr. Akizuki's patients were given a diet of brown rice, miso and soy sauce soup, seaweed (also know as sea vegetables), regular vegetables, and sea salt. He forbade any sugar consumption. Unlike most victims of the bomb's radiation, all of Dr. Akizuki's patients survived. He also saved himself: "This dietary method made it possible for me to remain alive and go on working vigorously as a doctor. The radioactivity may not have been a fatal dose, but thanks to this method, Brother Iwanaga, Reverend Noguchi, Chief Nurse Miss Murai, other staff members and in-patients, as well as myself, all kept on living in the lethal ashes of the bombed ruins."[17] This statement, made in 1980, testifies to a long life of recovery. The anecdotal evidence about relieving radiation effects following World War II is bolstered by more recent scientific studies done in Japan and other countries.

For example, Kazumitsu Watanabe, professor of cancer and radiation at Hiroshima University's atomic bomb research center, reports that when miso soup is eaten regularly, people may be more resistant to the ill effects of radiation. He studied small-intestine cells of mice—an area vulnerable to radiation, as seen in the high rates of nausea and diarrhea in bomb-vicinity victims and in cancer patients undergoing radiation therapy. As amusing as it is to imagine mice ingesting miso soup, it did protect them against high exposure X rays. Even when X rays at levels lethal to humans were administered to the mice, 60 percent survived, as opposed to 9 percent of the mice not fed miso. Professor Watanabe concluded that since the small intestines of humans and mice are similar, the favorable results for mice are relevant for humans as well.[18] I would rather the tests had been done on people already ill and in need of help instead of on mice, who could happily have lived without the X rays or the miso, but the evidence is intriguing. Ongoing tests at Hiroshima University show that the fermented miso helps eliminate radiation in the body. Akihiro Ito, head of one of the research medical teams, found that one way the fallout from nuclear and radioactive wastes is removed by miso is through stimulation of the circulatory and metabolic systems.[19] This is not to suggest that miso soup is the answer to nuclear disaster or that it will cure all cancers. Rather, an abundance of anecdotal evidence bolstered by a few promising studies makes it at least something we should know about. After all, we've adapted so many useful, thoroughly researched, well-made items from the Japanese, from cars to computers, why not potentially lifesaving medical findings?

Canadians, as well as the Japanese, have done suggestive research on seaweed and detoxifying the body. Stanley Skoryna, a physician at McGill University in Montreal, conducted animal studies showing that kelp reduced radioactive strontium absorbed through the intestines by

50 to 80 percent. Sodium alginate from brown algae (kombu is a good source) allowed the beneficial calcium to be absorbed through the intestines while simultaneously adhering to the strontium, taking it out of the body.[20] In other words, seaweed doesn't strip the body of what it needs; vitamins and minerals are left intact. It's the foreign substances, the toxic effects, that are removed. Studies done on radiation in the bones showed similar results: "The evaluation of biological activity of different marine algae is important because of their practical significance in preventing absorption of radioactive products of atomic fission as well as in their use as possible natural decontaminators. . . . The active alginates [seaweeds] also enhance the rat's normal physiological discrimination."[21] The same research team reported in a subsequent article that these findings have been "confirmed in other animals and in humans."[22]

No one Drew consulted in the alternative health field suggested that he reject radiation or surgery in favor of miso soup or sea vegetables. It was too late for that. His entire person was under assault, first from cancer, and later from surgery and intensive radiation. We all hoped fervently that the high-tech treatments would save his life. Miso soup and diet only provided an avenue to soothe the battlefield his body had become. Regardless of the length of his life, the day-to-day quality was improved. He felt great. In our new moment-to-moment mentality this was enough. To see Drew feeling so well was a gift we all enjoyed.

There was one catch here. Drew hated miso soup and sea vegetables. He might be able to answer "seaweed" with a wry grin to his fellow patients' questions, but seaweed was not his favorite food. I coaxed, wheedled, encouraged, and poured it down him.

Miso soup with seaweed shavings and tofu are not that unfamiliar to Americans. Japanese restaurants serve it routinely before meals. Because of volume, restaurants usually have to overcook and pre-prepare the miso soup, sacrificing some of its healthy properties, but it tastes the same—delicious to me, dreadful to Drew. At first I tried to make it tasty. I snipped the seaweed to a nearly tasteless powder and added his favorite vegetables. I made a rich, steaming bowl of thick, stewlike soup. He hated it. But he had seen the studies—he wanted to have it; he just didn't like it. Best that he treat it like a medicine, he decided. If the seaweed was shredded, the water-to-miso ratio reduced, and nothing added, he could drink it down quickly once it was lukewarm. (Add 1 teaspoon hacho or barley miso to $\frac{3}{4}$ cup warming water with $\frac{1}{2}$ inch finely shredded kombu or wakame seaweed. Cook for 2 to 3 minutes; never boil.)* This he didn't mind. It wasn't as bad as everything else he was putting up with. One more medicine—that he could tolerate.

There were new foods and old foods fixed in new ways he liked. Evelyne had prescribed a strictly Kushi Institute macrobiotic diet for cancer. Today if you talk to people eating macrobiotically, there is tremendous variety. Within some basic tenets, in time people settle into an assortment of foods that suits them. A macrobiotic diet is not the rigid schema of the early 1970s. However, with a healing diet, especially for cancer, strictness is advised. Each healing diet is prescribed uniquely, depending on the counselor and the ill individual, but it has a small circumference. At age forty-five, if I had been Drew, I would have adhered exactly to the recommended regimen. First, I had already experienced some great results. Second, I had studied or met people who had survived terminal cancers through macrobiotics. But Drew was twenty-one. He was taking my word for it. He believed the research, but he had no personal affinity with it. He felt he had nothing to lose and a lot to gain. The decision to try a new way of eating was his. He was behind it, but did it have to be so narrow? My emotional response was a pleading, resounding yes. My intellectual response was to bend. My raw, desperate voice stayed home alone. We agreed to be flexible. Better that he do the diet in a sort of, kind of way than try to be too strict and give it all up.

The beans and grains were not problems. I mashed pinto beans into look-alike, taste-alike refried beans without the oil, rolled them in warm 100 percent pure corn tortillas, and topped them with some fresh cilantro, a spray of fresh lime juice, and chopped scallions. Yum.

Brown rice fried in a touch of olive oil and tamari, with finely chopped colorful vegetables, was another hit. Quesadillas made with the same corn tortillas and soy mozzarella dairy-free cheese got a rave review. I admit to treachery here. I fixed the quesadillas without revealing the soy rather than regular cheese. I told Drew I had a treat for him. When he loved it but worried about eating cheese, I giggled and danced around the kitchen, revealing my sneakiness. He agreed he couldn't tell the difference. He was later to successfully pull the same trick on friends. Regardless of how revolting soy mozzarella sounds, once melted it tastes great. Evelyne told Drew he should avoid oils, baked goods (tortillas) because they contribute to mucus buildup, and anything even remotely

*I always cook beans with 3–6 inches of kombu. The seaweed decreases gas in the beans and dissolves into the bean mixture, tasteless and undetected by Drew.

processed (soy cheese) because it is harder to digest. The goal was to increase nutrients by using foods that would create the least amount of digestive work. The theories made sense to me. The reality, however, was that if Drew was craving cheese, better that he eat a chemical-free soy cheese from the health food store than dairy cheese, which could strain his system and contribute more heavily to mucus buildup in his sinus area, the area most in need of healing. Drew was also missing eggs, another heavy mucus food. Although tofu was not his favorite food, there is a way of scrambling it that looks like eggs and somehow satisfies like eggs. Leftover diced potatoes are fried with onions, crumbled tofu, and one-half teaspoon of turmeric (to make it all yellow). I also throw in a handful of chopped parsley to offset the small amount of forbidden oil and the frowned upon potatoes (too acidic). The taste is different from scrambled eggs but good, the color and texture similar. If I could continue to find substitutions for foods Drew missed, it would be easier. I was no longer worried he would revert to ice cream and pizza—he liked the new foods well enough and felt too good—but the easier it was to avoid the temptation, the better. One problem down, a new one around the corner.

As he felt better, he missed sweets. There is nothing as persistent as a sweet craving. But sweets, given the Hiroshima stories as well as the newer evidence about sugar and health, were a big deviation. Even fruit was not encouraged at this point. Drew didn't want fruit anyway. He wanted a real sweet. He wanted a chocolate eclair. We talked. He ate some sweets. Some nutritionists say that when you've been away from an unhealthy food it's good to try it again. You won't like it so much, and you can lay that fantasy to rest. Drew ate a candy bar. He loved it. It was just as delicious as he thought it would be. But he didn't feel great after eating it. His body was cleaned out and used to healthy foods. It was letting him know what he needed and what he didn't. So we plotted sweet foods that wouldn't make him tired. I made sweet potato pie: whole-wheat crust from the health food store, mashed and whipped red garnet yams (very rich and sweet), a touch of kuzu for thickener. Stephen, a tagalong on all of this, agreed it tasted like dessert.

Fruit jams (all fruit, all organic) spread on whole-wheat sourdough bread also did the trick: peach jam, raspberry spread, blueberry jelly—not recommended but better than Mars bars and satisfying, without the afterkick of energy loss.

Vegetables were also important. A lot of them he liked. Root vegetable casserole (winter sweet squash, rutabaga, turnip, onion, carrot, baked at 400 degrees for 1½ hours with garlic, shallots, olive oil, and fresh rosemary) was easy. What's called "cooked salad" was always a hit. In a large pot of boiling water, vegetables are cooked one or two minutes individually to make a brightly colored, crunchy array for the dinner table. Carrots, broccoli, pea pods, and beets, artfully arranged with a touch of tahini sauce (a Middle Eastern food made with ground sesame seeds, garlic, and lemon, often sold in grocery stores as humus) is one example. Leafy greens were more difficult. Slightly cooked, they are considered crucial. They provide rich minerals and vitamins and clean the liver, the recipient and sifter of all that comes into the body. (Pregnant women are today advised not to eat beef or chicken livers because they are so high in the chemicals and drugs fed to livestock.) Sometimes Drew found the greens more tolerable if finely chopped, stir-fried with other vegetables, or hidden in thick (non-miso) soups. Other times, when I was too tired, I just steamed them; and he downed them as he did miso soup—as a medicine, not a part of dinner.

Boston, an easy place in which to effect these changes, offers an excellent health food store chain* and many independent neighborhood stores, all selling organic produce, healthy staples, and a rich diversity of tasty foods, some prepared. Until you get used to it, this way of eating is labor-intensive, and thus prepared foods, if available, are a great help. We always had an array of snack foods, prepared fresh soups, excellent fish, lightly dressed salads made from grains, beans, and vegetables from the local health food store. Thus, despite what it sounds like, we didn't have to think about food preparation all of the time. I go into this level of detail only to show that with patience and open-mindedness, guidance and encouragement, even a young, American-fed college student can do what doctors tell Dr. Ornish that Americans can't do—change their eating habits to help save their lives. In fact, Drew felt I worried too much about taste and whether or not he liked the food. As I expected, the transition from college food, quintessential American cuisine with lots of sugar, spices, and animal products, was a tough one. Drew struggled with the decision to go on a healing diet, and he struggled to stay on it. But he reminded me that he had made the decision to do so and that he planned to stick with it, regardless of taste. After all, he was fighting for his life.

---

*An indication of growing consumer interest in health foods is the spectacular growth of natural food stores, such as Whole Foods Market, Inc., with chains of super markets in several parts of the country.

"Bring it on," he said. "Taste is not what's important here. It helps when it tastes good, but I'll eat dog food if you show me studies that it's good for cancer or radiation."

Dog food was not required. We made some adjustments, and Drew ate almost everything put in front of him.

I don't know if it would have been better for Drew to follow the diet more strictly. He doesn't either. Some counselors would say yes. He ate food that might encourage cancer regrowth. Some people have recovered from cancer on a macrobiotic diet, then relapsed when they reverted to their old eating habits. So some would say yes, it could be harmful, better to be strict at least temporarily, expanding carefully once well, adhering to the basic framework. Others might argue that each person must decide for himself or herself, as I felt. If Drew wanted a food so badly, perhaps some part of him needed it. In any case, he was the one who had to choose. He chose. He felt and looked well. He was doing fine with a strange diet. He was twenty-one, with cancer. Would I have done so well at that age? I doubt it.

In fact, he was doing exactly what Dr. R had recommended. He was eating a balanced diet—not exactly what Dr. R had in mind but indeed balanced. He was balancing the rest of his life, too: plenty of sleep, choosing social activities carefully, balancing rest and activity, facing what he could, avoiding what he didn't feel ready for. He was gaining weight and strength. He was becoming healthy again, healthier than he had been in over a year. He needed that strength to cope with the last phase of his treatment—the radiation.

While Drew was recovering in the hospital from the second surgery, Dr. R came and explained all of the details about the radiation. Radiation at any level, but particularly at the higher dosages, is a double-edged sword. Everyone knows that. The literature is full of both successes and failures. Some are saved by the radiation; some die from it. Some do both: they live longer, and the cancer is gone, but twenty years later they die of leukemia or another radiation-induced cancer.

Dr. R was the first doctor to use the word *cancer*. Andy pointed this out to him.

"I don't believe in euphemisms. If it's cancer, I call it cancer," Dr. R said gently.

He wasn't telling us anything we didn't know. He was, however, telling us something we hadn't fully faced, something we hadn't ourselves named. I started using the word first to myself, then occasionally to friends. Sally called after they had been home a few weeks.

"I find myself using the word *cancer* more often. It's like I'm trying it on, with caution. I'm getting used to it," she said.

Cancer. Why had it taken us all so long to use this word, to integrate its reality into our conversations even with ourselves? Was it the stigma, the fear of becoming leper-like in a culture that has trouble handling cancer—the word or the disease. I don't think so. I think what we all experienced was blind terror. Terror of emaciated children with wistful eyes in need of bone marrow transplants, of a truly malignant and malevolent disease possibly moving Drew toward death with excruciating, drawn-out pain. That is the image and for some the reality. By avoiding that word perhaps I was protecting Drew. I know I was protecting myself.

But one night, while we were watching TV, one of those public announcements for cancer research came on—a famous person, sounding serious, sincere, sappy, talking about personal experiences. Such messages didn't seem sappy anymore. Now I was the sap. I got tears in my eyes. Drew still hadn't spoken the word *cancer*. Was I being too evasive, avoiding the topic? In that far distance from reality, the classroom, I had advocated full disclosure to the ill. They had the right to know. I hadn't realized how complicated full disclosure to oneself, let alone the ill, was. Once I had started facing it in myself, however, I decided to wait for Drew to bring it up. He didn't. Somehow, while watching the TV, with Drew growing stronger, the treatment plan set, and the chances looking good, the moment seemed right. Later that night I said the word *cancer* while talking to Drew. He looked surprised.

"Do I really have cancer? I thought it was a gray area."

"No," I answered. "It's not a gray area. It's cancer. Remember Dr. R—he was the first to use the word."

Drew didn't remember. He hadn't heard. It had been stated loud and clear. All the rest of us remembered. Drew didn't. Cognition is remarkable. He obviously didn't want to hear it then. Still weak from the surgery, perhaps he couldn't yet cope with the C-word. Now he could. Somehow I knew this. He pursued the conversation. He was forthright, interested.

"How do you feel?" I asked, worried that he was worried.

"It'll be easier," he said. "I spend so much time trying to explain— grade 2, fuzzy area, sphenoid sinus. Now if people ask, I'll just say I have cancer—one word." He smiled.

He was so upbeat.

"What a guy," I laughed. "You even make me laugh talking about cancer."

Christiane Northrop, an obstetrician/gynecologist who works with women who have cancer, is right to trust her patients, especially if they exhibit the same unfailing sensibilities about recovery that Drew did. She writes:

Seven years ago I was eager to believe there was a right way and a wrong way to deal with cancer. I now find that I do not believe there is any one answer to the problem. . . . I have changed my approach to cancer; I no longer suggest one treatment modality over another. I refuse to decide for a given patient what treatment they should have for a given illness. Instead, I know that each person is fully capable, with some guidance, of choosing methods that will best enhance his or her healing process.[23]

I needed to remember this too. Don't push, I reminded myself. This is his life; he's protecting it well.

Dr. R went over the treatment plan in detail. He was optimistic. The people he was working with were doing well after five years. That was five years they might not have had without it.

In Drew's case, as in every case, he was working against a particular set of risks. Blindness and brain damage were the most frightening. Because the tumor had so bordered his brain and optic nerve, these would be the risk areas. I assumed that if this were to happen it would be instant. One day he would go in for treatment, and that day he might be blind. That could happen, Dr. R agreed, but it could happen in more complicated ways as well. In five, ten, thirty years, Drew could wake up blind or slowly going blind or gradually losing brain function. It could happen any time for the rest of his life. A cloud filled the room. It wasn't a dense cloud—all of these were just possibilities—but it was a pervasive cloud, a cloud that could hover just over your shoulder forever, a cloud that would get darker when a name couldn't be recalled, a headache appeared, or tired eyes made it harder to read. Once again uncertainty loomed. No definites here, only endless unknowns.

It seemed all the more pressing that everything possible be done to boost Drew's immune system, by now weak from the cancer and the surgeries, soon to be weaker when hit by megatons of proton beam radiation five days a week for eight weeks. His body also needed help in eliminating all of the toxins accrued from the disease as well as the cures. Dr. R explained that Drew would be receiving all of the radiation he could ever be given. If the tumor were to come back or another cancer appear, he could never again have radiation. This was one high-stakes game. But we were going for broke. Jean Craig, in her haunting story of losing two husbands—one to heart disease and one to cancer—bemoans the fact that neither she nor they knew anything about alternative therapies.[24] Drew was more fortunate. He would depend on the experts, Western heroic medicine doing what it does best, with all of the high tech, the warrior mentality of big guns against big enemies. And he would supplement that with the gentler, more Eastern route, continuing with visualization, acupuncture, and nutrition. We all hoped the blend would weigh the odds in Drew's favor.

Chapter Six

WESTERN REFLECTIONS ON EASTERN MEDICINE

In the fall of 1992, "The CBS Evening News" ran a five-part series on alternative medicines. The subject matter, increasingly in the news, is not unusual, but CBS's respectful treatment of these innovative methods is surprising. Acupuncture and relaxation, hypnotherapy and herbal remedies, chiropractics and macrobiotics were all investigated. Although no claims to absolute proof were made, the commentators expressed enthusiasm for success stories and preliminary data. Edie Magnus, the reporter covering the series, introduced the week with the statement "Proven or not, alternative treatments are now being used by more than half of all Americans, so conventional medicine finds itself forced to consider the unconventional."[1] And in concluding: "It seems the medical profession is learning to never say never."[2]

Similarly, in the spring of 1993, PBS ran the phenomenally popular series "Healing and the Mind," hosted by Bill Moyers. Acupuncture, herbal remedies, therapeutic support groups, biofeedback, visualizations, and more were reviewed through Moyers's own fascinated eyes. Experts and studies were quoted, and although it was made clear that no one has all of the answers, the obvious message was that to ignore such offerings meant mistaken medicine. The success of the series was followed by best-seller sales of the program's complementary book.[3] Concurrently, popular magazines such as *Time* and *Consumer Reports*, as well as MIT's *Technology Review*, ran favorable articles on new ways of expanding our understanding of health and healing.[4]

Such popularity shouldn't surprise us. After all, according to an article in the *New England Journal of Medicine*, many of us have sought help from a variety of nonmainstream providers. One in three respondents in a study of 1,539 adults in the United States "reported using at least one unconventional therapy in the past year, and one-third of these saw providers for unconventional therapy" (an average of 19 visits each).[5]

Given this growing interest, the call by Ralph W. Moss (editor of *Cancer Chronicles* and author of various books on health care) for more research on alternatives continues to be timely. He claims we need to weed out the useful from the false, the helpers from the harmers. The stakes are too high not to widen our visions and definitions.

. . . the continuing failure of orthodox medicine to deal satisfactorily with the major forms of cancer guarantees the growth of nonconventional approaches. Some of these approaches are possibly fraudulent or even harmful; others are doubtlessly inert. Yet among them all may well be some methods of great benefit to cancer patients. It is the job of the true scientist . . . to take a serious and open-minded look at all methods and claims. . . . A million new cases [of cancer] a year demand no less.[6]

The alternative methods used by Drew—especially acupuncture, relaxation techniques, and macrobiotics—though still considered exotic (particularly by him) are not so uncommon. Numerous stories and some studies suggest, amid controversy, that combining Eastern with Western medicines may be good for your health. Drew thought so. He felt that exactly the remedies now seeping into mass media discussions had helped him to help himself, to heal faster and feel better in the process.

Nutrition and Cancer

I met Rachel at my first natural-foods cooking class in 1991. A trim, elegant woman in her late fifties, dressed in a stylish jogging suit, her head wrapped in a silk turban, she looked like someone who would be whipping up nouvelle this or that, not studying healthy cooking.

"What brought you here?" I asked, looking for reassurance that I wasn't joining a cult of brown rice grazers.

"Cancer," she replied.

She had started with surgery, moving on to chemotherapy.

"When the doctors told me the cancer was still there, that it was spreading, and they couldn't do anything more, I figured what's to lose."

Rachel had read an article years before about people curing themselves of cancer with diet and had filed it away in the back of her mind. She'd been on a healing foods diet for about six months when I met her. Soon after starting she felt better than she had for some time. She traveled with her husband and kept up her busy social life, taking her own dinner to elegant dinner parties.

"I put my dinner in a lovely casserole and ask whoever's in the kitchen to warm it in the oven for me.

"Really? What are people's reactions?" I asked.

"Well, if they're close friends, it's understood; if not, I tell them in advance. What are they going to say? Besides people don't like to talk about cancer. They don't inquire past the word."

Rachel, like many seemingly self-cured cancer recoverers, is someone who believed in modern medicine. Like everyone I've talked to or read about, she learned of her illness from a doctor. In Rachel's case she did what they told her to do; it didn't work. There was nothing more medicine could offer. She was considered terminal. Ann Fawcett and Cynthia Smith's book *Cancer Free* includes numerous personal stories similar to Rachel's. Kit Kitatani, for example, underwent surgery for stomach cancer. The surgery was followed by chemotherapy. The cancer was still there, along with a new problem: bone marrow damage from the chemotherapy. When the doctor explained that he had nothing more to offer, Mr. Kitatani was furious.

"Don't be silly. You can't just drop me like this. Isn't there anything you can do?"

"Nothing," replied the doctor.[7]

Mr. Kitatani was lucky to run into a friend who claimed she had cured herself of terminal cancer with macrobiotics. He tried it. Seven years later, recovered, Mr. Kitatani is still a development specialist with the United Nations. He has used his influence to form the International Macrobiotic Society of the United Nations, introducing health information to agencies around the world.

A more famous example is Anthony Sattilaro, chief executive officer of Methodist Hospital in Philadelphia. A conventional doctor and administrator, after learning that he had metastasized prostate cancer, he turned to the best modern medicine had to offer. It was, after all, just down the hall from his office. But nothing worked for him, either. He was planning his funeral when he learned about macrobiotics from two hitchhikers. He never let go of medicine, clinging to bone scan results and consulting his team of specialists regularly. He would have gone the full medical course had it offered him the hope of a cure. But it hadn't. So, continuing to discuss his alternative path with skeptical doctors, he found help elsewhere.[8]

Rachel, Kit Kitatani, and Anthony Sattilaro did not reject modern medicine. Modern medicine rejected them. They are examples of one way that people happen upon an alternative route. Equally common in the literature are people who start out on the conventional route, reject it at varying points, and introduce their own game plan. They are, for the most part, conventional people who accepted their doctors' diagnoses and treatments. But somewhere along the way they lose faith; the cure is worse than the cancer, or the odds are so slim, the remedies so drastic, it doesn't seem worth it.

When Michael Shanik, in his early forties, was told he had a malignant melanoma, he and his wife did some research. His chances of survival, whether treated or not, were between 10 and 20 percent. The Shaniks discovered macrobiotics, changed their diet, slowed down their lives, and, over the strenuous objections of their physician, turned down the suggested surgery. Mr. Shanik received a chilling letter from his doctor: "I need for you to be aware of the high risk you're taking by choosing your present course of action, which appears limited to using a macrobiotic diet. I trust that I have made myself clear."

To Mr. Shanik, "it was like receiving a death notice." After agonizing considerations he decided to stay with the diet. "We were unsure of macrobiotics because we didn't know much about it. One thing we were sure of though was that Michael's chances were slim to none, according to the doctors, where macrobiotics offered us some hope," his wife Mickey recalls.[9]

Michael Shanik thinks he made the right choice. Today he has no diagnosable cancer. He feels terrific.

A third, smaller group rejects medicine altogether. Dirk Benedict, the TV and film star, in his *Confessions of a Kamikaze Cowboy*, takes the solitary wrangler approach. A Montana boy, steeped in all the American

West loner trappings, he rides off to Michio Kushi's remote New Hampshire cabin, with only his miso soup and a few other sundries, to tough it out—alone. Tough it out he does. He, unlike Dr. Sattilaro, has no use for doctors and their "shot in the dark" approach to illness in general, his prostate cancer in particular. Unlike Dr. Sattilaro, who is careful to commend modern medicine despite its inability in his case to save his life, Benedict launches tirades against the whole profession: "There's an old saying that goes, 'The only two things you can't escape are death and taxes.' I disagree. The only two things you can't escape are death and doctors! And if you have enough to do with the latter, you increase your chances of the former."[10] But escape death and doctors he does. At least this time around.

Like the other riveting and inspiring stories in print, from such sources as Ann Fawcett and Cynthia Smith's book to individual accounts like Elaine Nussbaum's *Recovery* and Anthony Sattilaro's *Recalled by Life*, the prognosis is promising. The data, although anecdotal, are ample enough to warrant attention and more scientific study.

Drew's story is different. Unlike the survivors described above, he stayed with conventional medicine. Western techniques of surgery and radiation played the biggest part in his recovery. Unlike the other cases, no one suggested that Drew forgo the recommended procedures and rely solely on macrobiotics. I wanted them to. It's not that Drew would have done so or that I would have urged him to. But I craved the reassurance of "Oh that, yes I've seen that a lot; people recover without surgery or radiation. My friend X is just fine." That would have been comforting, less serious. No one said anything of the sort. No one in any field claims everyone can be cured of cancer. Macrobiotic counselors are no exception. Anthony Sattilaro reports that Michio Kushi, when confronted with people who seemed past hope, would say, "It is very difficult. We won't know for a few months."[11]

At a dinner in honor of Herman Aihara, probably in his early seventies and considered one of the great macrobiotic theorists and practitioners in this country, along with Michio Kushi, I got this same message. My friend Karin told him about Drew. What did he think? He looked at me sadly.

"Very serious," he said and then looked down.

I felt the conversation was over. Karin persisted.

"He's had the first surgery. The second is scheduled for next week."

"Yes, of course he must have the surgery," agreed Mr. Aihara.

What! Of course he must have the surgery? This from a man who had devoted his life to curing the incurable, fixing the unfixable through macrobiotics. Mr. Aihara wanted to eat his dinner; he was at a party. I wanted a miracle. I wanted macrobiotics, at least in theory, to be that miracle. I knew we would not reject Dr. T's advice, but I wanted Mr. Aihara to reject it. He wouldn't either.

Just as Drew did not reject medical science, the doctors did not reject him. They were cautiously optimistic. The word *terminal* was never used; the procedures were based on successful results. The statistics, the same old 1 percent odds (now 5 percent) that had let us down repeatedly, were still being pulled out to give reassurance. We let them. But not completely. After all, we, like the people whose case studies I had read, were trying a variety of other modalities. But we weren't taking an either/or approach. We were hoping West would meet East, that they would complement each other, one technique bolstering another. We were combining what Hugh Faulkner calls "complementary [alternative] medicines" with orthodox (conventional) medicine.

Hugh Faulkner, a retired English doctor, was diagnosed in 1987 with pancreatic cancer. Firmly entrenched in the medical model, he followed his doctor's advice.

"When Marian [his wife], assuming that I had a cancer which was likely to be inoperable, asked what would happen if I didn't have the operation, Mr. Cochrane said that I would almost certainly obstruct. Naturally I decided to have the operation."[12]

Despite all that could be done, Dr. Faulkner knew his chances were slim. Pancreatic cancer, on the increase, is considered inevitably fatal. In a study of 196 cases, done at Yale, the average survival was seven months. One person lived six years. All died.

Dr. Faulkner had the surgery. He also had shiatsu massage and started a macrobiotic diet. Today he feels well and continues to work in retirement on what interests him most, health care and writing about his own cancer experience.[13] He sums up his situation as follows:

Today, well over two years after the initial diagnosis, I feel extremely well. I can't claim conclusively that my cancer is regressing, though ultrasound and a CAT scan suggest some shrinking and liquefaction in the center of the tumor area. Nor can I prove that my present state is the result of macrobiotics. This story is just another example of the anecdotal accounts that many physicians quite properly find unconvincing. However, it has persuaded me that further dialogue is desirable between orthodox Western medical science and complementary medicine. The situation in the United States where both sides appear to hurl insults at one another across a Berlin Wall of misunderstanding is deplorable.[14]

Dr. Faulkner is right; his story is an anecdote, not something to base a medical practice on. He's also right that this should not stand in the way of further dialogue. And perhaps this metaphorical Berlin Wall is crumbling, just as the real one did. There are, in fact, many intriguing studies that help this dialogue. In earlier chapters I discussed studies on radiation and diet as well as a growing literature on nutrition and general health. The studies I list in this chapter, the ones directly related to cancer and its possible cure and prevention, were the ones that Drew found most convincing. And he, like everyone else with cancer who turns to alternatives, needed to be convinced.

Drew may not love leafy greens or brown algae in his soup, but the more he read, the more he too was intrigued. He stopped saying "there's nothing to lose" and started talking about all there was to gain.

The growing use of alternative medicines by so many people is perhaps easier to understand once cancer statistics in America are considered. According to the American Cancer Society one in three Americans alive today "will eventually have cancer." The National Cancer Institute figures show that between 1988 and 1990 lifetime *risk* for developing cancer (of any kind) was 42.5 percent for men, 38.8 percent for women. Between 1973 and 1990, cancer *rates* rose 18.3 percent.[15]

Of those afflicted, only roughly one in three survive, the same survival rate as in 1950. Furthermore, Dr. Steven A. Rosenberg of the National Cancer Institute, while applauding modern medical techniques in the treatment of some cancers, concludes: "Except possibly in selected patients with cancer of the stomach, there has been no demonstrated improvement in the survival of patients with the ten most common cancers when radiation therapy, chemotherapy, or both have been added to surgical resection."[16] In fact, these therapies can wreak damage from toxic effects.

Far from winning the "war on cancer," other reports, such as one by John Cairns of the Harvard School of Public Health, show heavy losses: "[A]part from the success with Hodgkin's disease, childhood leukemia and a few other cancers, it is not possible to detect any sudden change in death rates for any of the major cancers that could be credited to chemotherapy."[17] And John C. Bailar, who has worked for the National Cancer Institute and the *New England Journal of Medicine* and currently holds a faculty position at McGill University, told the President's cancer panel, "Whatever we have been doing, it is not working."[18]

With newer radiation techniques, greater precision in the use of chemotherapy, and better understanding of mutations in the chemical makeup of genes, some argue that these statistics are improving. I hope so, Drew certainly hopes so, but more time is needed to know. It's no wonder Americans find cancer the most frightening disease around.

But if these statistics overwhelm and frighten, others offer hope. As early as 1964, the World Health Organization stated that cancer could be 80 percent preventable with dietary and life-style changes. More recently, a few cancer specialists have been calling for a change in emphasis from cure to prevention. John C. Bailar and Elaine M. Smith write: "[W]e are losing the war against cancer, notwithstanding progress against several uncommon forms of the disease. . . . A shift in research emphasis, from research on treatment to research on prevention, seems necessary if substantial progress against cancer is to be forthcoming."[19] John Cairns too, in *Scientific American*, calls for prevention, citing history as our teacher. Historically, all of our major public health problems, from smallpox to tuberculosis to polio, have been overcome with prevention, not after-the-fact treatments.

In the absence of a vaccine against cancer, the emphasis on prevention is primarily on nutritional and life-style changes. Most dietary recommendations are similar to a macrobiotic diet—increase whole grains and vegetables, decrease animal fats and sweets, eat fresh, nonprocessed foods. A decrease in fats and chemicals especially increases health. Toxic chemicals are stored in fats in the body; thus, a diet high in both presents a double liability. (Since breast tissue is so high in fat, perhaps the escalating use of chemicals and of breast cancer rates are related.)

Despite the call for prevention from many medical experts and promising news on a variety of alternative approaches, some in medicine cry quackery at anything that veers from conventional treatment. Some of these dissenters find the public's interest in alternatives disturbing. The cited concerns of lack of proof, the proliferation of strange remedies that hark back to snake oils, and a fear that the public, even when well educated, is too gullible* all raise legitimate questions. But the answer to these questions is to fund research to study new popular methods, not to dismiss them. Orthodox understandings must include what the public clearly wants and is pursuing, often in the face of dashed hopes by conventional cures.

Today new studies are being done on alternative medicines. National centers like the National Institutes of Health and the American Cancer Society, as well as medical centers around the country, are slowly opening their research agendas to include prevention and innovative medicines. But completed studies that meet scientific criteria are not yet common. Studies in progress may be promising but are rarely or only recently publicized. However, when a study with negative results is done, it is heralded as a landmark, proof that danger lurks in *all* "unproven" techniques, not just the one researched. (Victor Herbert, for example, lumps together and blasts what he terms "lucrative holistic practices" from "acupuncture to iridology, chiropractics, homeopathy, holistic psychotherapy . . . [to] therapeutic touch, and the hazards of herbal medicine.")[20]

The much noted study by Barrie R. Cassileth and colleagues received lavish attention.[21] Cassileth's elegantly designed research compares seventy-eight advanced cancer patients undergoing conventional treatments with seventy-eight similar patients participating in an alternative program at a center in San Diego, California. This center dispensed a mostly raw-foods diet, injections of bacille Calmette-Guerin and an immunity-enhancing vaccine, and coffee enemas. (Some participants at the alternative center were also using conventional treatments.) No differences were found in lengths of survival between the two groups. The San Diego group reported a decreased quality of life based on factors such as feelings of hunger (no doubt a result of a diet of raw foods).

Subsequent articles have used this study as a warning siren against "unproven" methods of cancer treatment[22] (a warning that assumes incorrectly that conventional always means proven). Actually, this study

---

*The majority of people using alternative medicines are likely to be well educated, a fact that puzzles critics of unorthodox procedures. There is no mystery here, however. Well-educated people are more likely to have the resources to pursue treatments that are not covered by private insurance or public funding. The two-tiered health care system in the United States, where the haves get the best and the have-nots don't, applies to alternative care as well.

merely shows that people receiving care at one specialized alternative center fared no better (and in terms of length of survival, no worse) than those undergoing routine treatments. To generalize from this study (unless the same alternative procedures are used) is misleading and unscientific.

The most startling implication of this study, however, goes unmentioned in the reporting article, the subsequent citations, and the popular press: To find no differences in length of survival between those receiving conventional therapies and those receiving coffee enemas seems extraordinary to me and as telling about the former modes of treatment as the latter.

The macrobiotic diet (not included in the above-mentioned programs) also seems to strike a negative chord in some areas of medicine. Like my own first mistaken assumptions, articles against macrobiotics assume that the diet is rigidly brown-rice-dominated. Cassileth and Berlyne, in another article warning against alternative therapies, incorrectly claim that a macrobiotic diet "includes only whole grains, some specially cooked vegetables, and miso."[23] In 1984 the American Cancer Society cautioned, "The more restrictive macrobiotic diets pose a serious hazard to health."[24] And in *Oncology Nursing Forum*, nurses are told to counsel cancer patients away from macrobiotics to avoid nutritional deficiencies.[25] Despite lack of data to support such warnings, valid concerns do emerge from the articles. Macrobiotics has not been systematically studied, with proper controls and conclusions.* But just as yet no studies definitively prove macrobiotics works, none proves it doesn't. *All* cancer therapies, conventional and alternative, need more rigorous study. The current evidence for macrobiotics is largely personal testimony with some suggestive studies on foods included in the diet. More research is needed. The second concern is that macrobiotics can lead to nutritional deficiencies (for example, the vitamin B's and iron) in those most at risk from such a lack—the ill. This is a danger. As with any new food regimen, especially one that is exotic to the preparer, great care must be taken. Grains, beans, nuts, and seeds should be combined to create enough complementary proteins. It is also important to include fish (twice a week was recommended for Drew) and daily servings of sea

---

*This is changing. The National Institutes of Health has awarded a research grant to study macrobiotics and cancer. Lawrence Kushi, Sc.D., an epidemiologist at the University of Minnesota School of Public Health, is principal investigator. He will conduct the research with a team of doctors, nutritionists, and fellow scientists.

vegetables to ensure that minerals and vitamins are sufficiently provided. Finally, consumers of all health care need to find qualified practitioners to guide them, and macrobiotics is no exception. We should ask a lot of questions, take nothing on faith, call umbrella organizations for referrals, ask to speak to others who have tried suggested programs. Demand to be convinced before accepting advice from any consultant, whether conventional or alternative.

Despite the critics, a congressional publication on health and long-term care supports the view that a careful macrobiotic diet is nutritionally sound.

... the current macrobiotic diet ... appears to be nutritionally adequate if the mix of foods proposed in the dietary recommendations is followed carefully. There is no apparent evidence of any nutritional deficiencies among macrobiotic practices. The diet is consistent with the recently released dietary guidelines of the National Academy of Sciences and the American Cancer Society in regard to possible reduction of cancer risks.[26]

And Michael Lerner, in a review (and careful critique) of Cassileth and Berlyne's article (both appeared in the same issue of *Oncology*) suggests that "engaging in health-promoting behaviors may improve general health and functional status, which are sometimes associated with better outcomes in cancer. There are frequently benefits in terms of quality of life. ... Improvement in quality of life in cancer is, after all, of extraordinary significance in itself."[27] Lerner includes in his long list of "health promoting behaviors" the remedies Drew found so beneficial: Chinese medicine such as acupuncture, relaxation exercises, and a balanced vegetarian diet.

Controversy over macrobiotics, still evident, is nonetheless decreasing. As noted doctors such as Dean Ornish and Benjamin Spock speak on it at conferences, as dietary changes are increasingly recommended, macrobiotics—perhaps not always labeled as such—becomes more acceptable, at least in theory.

As the emphasis begins to shift to prevention through individual life-style changes, I would argue again that responsibility extends out from the individual to the environment and society for prevention. Once someone is ill, however, cure is an individual road. Drew didn't have time to work on cleaning up the smoggy air or polluted waters of New England as a means to rid himself of a malignant tumor—that's something for him to think about when well. But he could change his own care and work on his own cleanup. The available evidence suggested that he would be foolish not to. There are no nutritional studies of chondrosarcoma, grade 2, under the optic chiasm in the sphenoid sinus. In fact, there are probably not enough people in the world in this category to study it. But other studies focusing on other cancers are useful.

Breast cancer struck one in twenty American women in 1940, one in eleven in 1981, one in eight today, and is still rising. In Massachusetts, where it is declared an epidemic, breast cancer rose 26 percent between 1982 and 1988.[28] Once considered a disease of older women, usually postmenopause, today it strikes all ages.

Controversy rages over whether fats in the diet and/or estrogens accumulated in the body encourage breast cancer. Studies done on people, difficult to control, show conflicting results about a fat/fiber component in the cause of this disease.[29] Even those most critical of the diet/breast cancer link, however, recommend that women adhere to a low-fat diet to prevent other cancers, such as cancer of the colon, as well as heart disease.

More numerous are the laboratory animal studies. Rats injected with mammary cancer fared better with a high-fiber diet,[30] miso soup,[31] and sea vegetables.[32] A recent University of Wisconsin study linked fermented soy sauce (on the same principle as miso soup) to reduced chances of stomach cancer.[33] The connections go on and on. Colon, lung, esophageal, ovarian, and stomach cancers, leukemia, and lymphoma have all been linked to diet. The same basic habits seem to apply— the more fiber in the form of fresh vegetables and grains and the fewer animal products such as dairy and meats, the better. If you throw in some fish, beans, and, if you're adventurous, tofu (shown to help prevent stomach cancer in a Japanese study[34]), your chances of preventing cancer or helping to cure it may increase.

Doctors have been slow to embrace disease/diet connections in general and cancer/diet linkages in particular. They are beginning to change. The evidence, although preliminary, is suggestive. Especially in the area of heart disease and fat, the news is everywhere. Cancer/food relationships are less understood and accepted, but evidence is growing. These studies, however tentative, are intriguing. But dietary change is difficult, and when it comes to such oddities as miso soup, tofu, or seaweeds, there is much resistance.

Vivien Newbold, a physician on the staff of Holy Redeemer Hospital in Philadelphia, wrote a paper on her study of six patients diagnosed with various advanced cancers, including metastasized pancreatic cancer and malignant melanoma. The common thread was that all underwent some conventional medical treatment and all were considered terminal. One woman died; the other five people did not. This story is as interesting for its politics as for its health news.

Newbold's paper is written in the form of case histories (six patients are too few for a formal study). Each person's case was deemed hopeless by her or his doctors. All six, however, adhered to a macrobiotic diet, individually tailored to their particular illness. The five who recovered are thriving after five years or more, with no sign of cancer. When one woman, apparently recovered, gave up macrobiotics, the cancer returned, and she died. She might have died anyway. Vivian Newbold at no time claims to have proved her case. Rather, she calls on the medical community to ask more questions, look more closely, do the studies that could provide more definite knowledge. Drawing on her own and other case studies, as well as preliminary controlled research, she concludes, "in view of the many remissions of cancer and other serious diseases that have occurred in connection with this alternative approach, the medical community would serve itself well to investigate these phenomena seriously."[35]

In the Office of Technology Assessment report *Unconventional Cancer Treatments*, a congressional investigator writes, "If cases such as Newbold's were presented in the medical literature, it might help stimulate interest among clinical investigators in conducting controlled prospective trials of macrobiotic regimens, which could provide valid data on effectiveness."[36] But the medical journals were *not* interested. No one would publish Newbold's work. She was told that the readership wouldn't find it interesting. Help in the endless, time-is-running-out, heavy-losses "war on cancer" not interesting to doctors?

Perhaps this is changing. In the summer of 1993, Newbold, with five other doctors, published a retrospective study on diet and cancer in the *Journal of the American College of Nutrition*. The authors suggest that a macrobiotic diet extended life and quality of life in a sample of people with pancreatic, prostate and other nutrition-related cancers. The authors call for more systematic research to follow up their own small study.[37] In the meantime more and more people are doing their own experiments—experiments on themselves. After all, as Drew kept saying as he held his nose and drank miso soup, "At least this stuff can't hurt me."

Visualizations and Cancer

Dr. Newbold is careful to point out that other alternative modalities are also important. The meditation and visualization exercises that Drew practiced before, during, and after the surgeries helped to keep him steady in the face of emotional and physical chaos. These techniques are also being researched. Once again, controversy abounds in this area. Even if connections among mind, body, and stress do exist, the relationship of these connections to actual illness, and possible benefits from meditation and relaxation exercises, are more uncertain.[38] Striving for scientific certainty, research units in hospitals all around the country are conducting studies on the usefulness of meditation and visualization for panic attacks, diabetes, multiple sclerosis, AIDS, heart disease, cancer, and other illnesses. Although behavioral medicine is still considered a fringe medical area, researchers like Herbert Benson and Jon Kabat-Zinn in Massachusetts, Martin Rossman in California, and Janice Kiecolt-Glaser and Ronald Glaser in Ohio are lending legitimacy to this field.

Jon Kabat-Zinn has gained acceptance by many mainstream practitioners with a relaxation video used in hospitals. At the University of Massachusetts Medical Center, where he runs a stress-reduction clinic, all inpatients are told about his video, which is shown on the hospital channel throughout the day. More than one hundred hospitals around the country currently offer this tape to patients in their rooms. One patient at New York University Medical Center wrote Kabat-Zinn about how much his voice had meant to her:

"[W]ords of yours have stayed with me through two frightening cancer surgeries. So many other comforting thoughts that you offer on your video have helped me keep my sanity. . . . So many other patients during my hospital stay were taking comfort from your voice. . . . I am still hurting from my most recent surgery, and I am still scared, but I have too many good, in fact wonderful, moments because of your help."[39]

Despite the growing awareness of the usefulness of relaxation techniques, no doctor we saw suggested that Drew could benefit from such exercises, and few people we knew were aware of them. As with macrobiotics, the gains could be enormous, but first we needed to learn about the techniques and potential benefits through our own review of the scientific literature.

No one working in the field of behavioral medicine claims conclusive proof. As in most of medicine, whether conventional or alternative, certainty is more elusive than we realize, and good research with steady results is hard to find. But a growing mixture of case studies, extensive clinical experience, and new scientific information on mind–nervous system–immune system connections is worth attention.

The relatively new field of psychoneuroimmunology is clearly examined by Steven Locke, of Harvard Medical School, in his book *The Healer Within*.[40] He explains the scientific findings on how white blood cells, crucial to immune function, receive messages from the brain through the nervous system. If the immune system is vital to identifying foreign matter in the body, whether it be a virus or a cancer cell, and the mind can influence that function in some way as yet not fully understood, then yet another avenue toward recovery is at least explorable.

Researchers have shown that immunity can fluctuate under stress. Medical students' "natural killer cells" (immune cells that kill viral cells) went down during exams and back up when the stress had passed.[41] Separation, divorce, loss, unemployment, and so forth have been shown to lower immunity. The central question here is whether lowered immunity leads to poorer health. Logically, one might say that of course it does, but to date there is no evidence that gives definite answers to these questions. In numerous studies, Janice Kiecolt-Glaser and Ronald Glaser show a relationship between stress and lowered immune function. They stop short, however, of asserting a correlation between these dynamics and the development or cure of diseases such as cancer. They don't deny the connections but argue for more research.[42] Others, such as Kabat-Zinn, have found emerging evidence that chronic stress and impaired immune function can lead to bodily breakdown, not as a single causal agent but as one possible factor among many.[43] They claim that visualizations can help to heal this breakdown.

It's not clear at what point meditating or visualizing changes patterns of stress, immune dysfunction, and the possibility of disease. If you do relaxation exercises regularly, perhaps bolstering your immunity, making stresses more manageable, will you avoid getting sick in the first place? Are these techniques good prevention against the ills of modern life? Can I avoid getting cancer if I keep myself calm in the face of whatever comes my way in the last years of this rather beat-up century? Or is it best applied as one of a series of solutions to illness once present? Can it help cure cancer or heart disease?

These questions probably pose too simple either-or scenarios that no two researchers or practitioners in the area would agree on. But meditations do seem to help people cope with a variety of problems, from day-to-day stress to heart disease. Jon Kabat-Zinn, focusing on healing and coping rather than curing, would argue that the ends don't matter; it's the means, the moment-to-momentness of life, that we need to concentrate on. He has people practice mindfulness, a focus on each second as important. If you live only another day, at least that day has been experienced to the fullest.

Dean Ornish, after working with cardiovascular patients in a more cure-oriented framework, argues that diet, walking, yoga, and meditation are crucial in the reversal of heart disease. The one man in his study who died ate the prescribed diet but insisted on too vigorous exercise, ferociously competing against the clock, ignoring the more meditative yoga exercises and the visualizations. In the PBS documentary on this study, Ornish suggests to this man that he work on relaxing, encouraging him to do more meditation and yoga exercises, to no avail. Ornish concludes, after the man's death, that the meditative skills must be emphasized, taught, and encouraged more strongly. Perhaps he would have died anyway. It's dangerous to generalize from one case, and not everyone can be cured or cure themselves all of the time. But the excellent results of the other participants, as opposed to degenerative conditions in the control group, which followed careful conventional heart association medical guidelines, are hopeful.

Hope is what Drew derived from these exercises. Whether stress is a factor in the cause of cancer or not, once you have cancer, it is inevitable. Hopelessness runs rampant. Control or any illusion of it is out the window. Relaxation exercises helped Drew counteract these sensations. They helped him sleep and feel less passive in the face of illness and the patient role. Visualizing the tumor shrinking, the cells healing and returning to normal, delivering his body back to him well and as he had known it, gave him a sense of hope. He was not helpless in the face of an unknown. He knew that tumor. The illness was his own, reclaimed from the pages of medical textbooks, taken back from the abstract categories mulled over in disease talk by his doctors. The unfamiliar became familiar. The foreign became part of him, a part he could recognize and work with. Fear decreased; confidence grew.

Perhaps these exercises improved his immune function. Perhaps they made him physically and psychologically stronger. Perhaps not.

What did happen was that he felt better from doing them, and when it comes to illness, feeling better is crucial. The images Drew used changed during the course of his illness. They always, however, involved gentle healers making his head glow with health.

A young, six-year-old boy with a tumor in his brain stem visualized a different scenario. His mother told me his story on the phone one day. Her son was uninterested in gentle healers. He sought high adventure with a crew of Ninja Turtles. His mother explained to me, "When he was diagnosed, we tried to remove violent images from his life, and so we were against his watching the Ninja Turtle videos. But in the hospital that's what he wanted to watch. And he watched them over and over. The Ninja Turtles became for him the good guys fighting the tumor."

Once home she found her four-year-old son and her ill six-year-old son dancing the "Ninja Turtle fighting the tumor" dance. She took this image, created by her son, and used it when guiding him through relaxation/visualization exercises.

She and I marveled at her son's insights into what he needed, his ability to create his own healing stories. It reminded us both, as caretakers, how important it is to listen to the person you're helping, how wise we all are about the choices we make to feel better, regardless of how young or how old.

Stress centers around the country, usually in hospitals, offer classes or programs to teach people how to cope with stress and live with illness. When these stress centers exist in hospitals, doctors become more aware of them, and many refer their patients. At the University of Massachusetts Hospital, the expected referrals for chronic pain occur regularly. Increasingly, however, even the more skeptical specialists, such as oncologists and cardiovascular physicians, recommend people. Some doctors, so impressed with the results, sign up for themselves.

There are excellent books, accompanied by audiotapes, available in bookstores and libraries. Authored by practitioners, many of whom are physicians, they offer a self-help approach if stress centers are too distant or costly (see Appendix B). None claims to be the only road, and all leave room for individual adjustment.

Kabat-Zinn's comprehensive book, with the ominous title *Full Catastrophe Living*, gives a detailed introduction to mind/body connections as well as the step-by-step, how-to approach taken in his stress-reduction clinic. He reminds us not to think of single causes and simple solutions. In his discussion of stress and the immune system he notes that larger forces can also be at work: "Of course it is possible for a person to be exposed to such massive levels of carcinogenic substances that even a healthy immune system would be overwhelmed . . . toxic dumping . . . Love Canal . . . Hiroshima, Nagasaki . . . Chernobyl. . . . In short, the development of any kind of cancer is a multistage, complex occurrence involving our genes and cellular processes, the environment, and our individual behavior and activities."[44]

Equally important in a growing literature that can be too simply interpreted, Kabat-Zinn debunks the idea of blaming the ill person for negative emotions. If we are to embrace alternative methods, it is crucial that they not be presented as a palliative for all of the supposedly bad things people did to themselves to get sick. Brain surgery should not be considered an antidote to negativity or overemotionalism. Mind-altering exercises shouldn't be either. In the controversy over whether bad thoughts, negative mind-sets, or personality types encourage disease, Kabat-Zinn doesn't take sides. Rather, he says it doesn't really matter. It's how the person is treated that matters.

Even if it turns out that there is a statistically important relationship between negative emotions and cancer [not shown to date], to suggest to a person with cancer that his or her disease was caused by psychological stress, unresolved conflict, or unexpressed emotions would be totally unjustified. It amounts to subtly or not so subtly blaming the person for his or her disease. . . . This attitude is far more likely to result in increased suffering than in healing.[45]

Not only is a blame-and-guilt cycle unjustified, it's illogical. The idea that certain personality types get cancer is ungrounded. One out of three Americans get cancer; are they all similar in character? I think not. Besides, babies get cancer. Dogs get cancer. Is this because of their negative emotions? Did they cause their illnesses? Seems unlikely. In any case, Drew used these exercises not to overcome negativity or to change his personality type, whatever that may be. He used them to relax, to feel better. To feel better. It's that simple.

Acupuncture and Cancer

There are many alternative approaches to disease available worldwide today that Drew did not try. To cite a few of the many respected healing methods used here and in other countries: First, the Queen of England employs a personal homeopathic doctor as well as an allopathic (conventional medicine) one. Second, Ayurvedic medicine, increasingly popular in the United States, is a healing method from India. Ayurvedic practice combines meditation, diet, herbs, minerals, and aromas to create balance, and thus health, in the individual and thus in nature. And third, Germany has a network of cancer rehabilitation health spas where all who have cancer can go for six-week stays, once a year for five years. The spas are located in mountainous settings, with all of the amenities of hotels combined with the medical care of hospitals. Diet and exercise are tailored to the individual with an emphasis on low-fat, natural foods. People on chemotherapy are given injections of vitamins and minerals to counteract side effects. Herbal remedies, massage, and spa baths are available to pamper the clientele, and people report feeling indulged and energized. It is a humane gesture to those with an inhumane disease. And it is free of charge as part of the national health plan.

Any of these approaches might have helped, but we didn't know much about them or they were not available to us and time was short. Drew relied on what those close to him already knew. Nutrition was the most known, experimented with, and thus focused on. Complementary to diet and relaxation exercises was acupuncture. Drew had no phobias about needles, and once reassured that it was not painful in the sense of shots all over the body (ultrathin disposable needles barely pierce the skin; blood is not drawn), he agreed to try it. After all, he said, once you've eaten seaweed, anything goes.

In her letters, Rebecca encouraged Drew by describing how ubiquitous acupuncture was in China. She found it to be the taken-for-granted treatment for a variety of ills and procedures. She reported that her professor of ancient Chinese history at the University of International Business and Economics in Beijing had undergone a cesarean birth with acupuncture as the sole anesthetic. She had felt no pain during the surgery, and at its end she got up from the operating table, picked up the baby, and walked home. Furthermore, my mother's and my own experiences pointed Drew toward acupuncture. Once again I was able to provide him with a broader data base to strengthen our anecdotal stories— data that rarely furnished precise, scientific verification but did offer suggestive evidence.

In the late 1980s I had introduced Chinese medicine as a topic in my medical sociology classes. I had become increasingly dissatisfied with the standard curriculum based on explorations of Western medicine, its definitions, strengths, and deficiencies. I decided to add readings and discussions of alternative visions of what health and illness meant in a variety of cultures. Students met lecturers on Chinese medicine with enthusiasm. The topic's foreignness opened their eyes to more diverse interpretations of other cultures as well as their own.

Acupuncture, like macrobiotics and relaxation therapies, through different means strives to correct imbalances, restoring equilibrium to a person, body, and mind. It is based on a complicated system of meridians and energy flows that run throughout the body. Chi, the vital energy, moves freely through those open meridians or pathways when all is well. Illness is understood as an imbalance in the meridian system. Energy may be blocked, deficient, or excessive, creating what is understood to be conditions of disharmony. Each person's pattern is unique. Acupuncture needles, when placed on specific points along the meridians, work to restore balance and vitality, thus health. Herbs are often prescribed in addition to acupuncture treatments. Philosophically, Chinese medicine is rooted in a balance between opposites that also blend into each other—yin and yang. As with macrobiotics, extremes in either direction swing one out of line. Careful work through food or pressure points is suggested to restore harmony.

This overly simplistic explanation is akin to explaining nuclear physics in a paragraph. Excellent books and articles abound that explain in more detail what is in fact difficult for the Western mind to grasp (see Appendix C), for one cannot see meridians, Chi, or pressure points under a microscope. Practitioners do not conduct extensive tests, lab workups, and so on. Rather, an acupuncturist will take all six pulses in each wrist, to assess the depth, pace, length, strength, and quality of each pulse as a means to consider organ health and energy flow. Practitioners will also observe facial color, examine the tongue for coatings, color, and so forth, and, like Western doctors, take a detailed history.

Acupuncture, widely practiced in the United States under regulations differing from state to state, is increasingly studied in hospitals by doctors. One source cites 6,500 accredited acupuncturists in the United States today, and many more are unregistered. Numerous schools of acupuncture exist throughout the country, with more in the making.[46] In Austria, acupuncture as well as homeopathy are now part of conventional medical training.

But in America much of the public finds acupuncture confusing. A friend in search of an acupuncturist for her debilitating carpal tunnel problems in both wrists reported, "It's not exactly easy to find a specialist here. It's not like I can look for the best acupuncturist in town to treat carpal tunnel syndrome. They don't use those terms. They're likely to think it's the liver or something."

Regardless of its strangeness to Westerners, however, people are going to acupuncturists in increasing numbers. It is U.S. medicine that remains the most skeptical. Despite acupuncture's growing acceptance in other countries and a three-thousand-year history in China, "Where's the proof?" is the most common question established medicine asks.

It may be a long time before these attitudes change. Scientific studies here and abroad are underway. Proof, as we understand it, is difficult, however. For example, if someone has colon cancer, in Western medicine you do tests and come up with a diagnosis. Surgery and chemotherapy can be done, and the person may live or die, but once you have a sufficient number of people—and there is no shortage here—you can try different dosages of a drug until it starts to work or fails. You can set up control groups, and you will learn what works, what doesn't. Over time, with enough rats or enough people, you may be able to show something conclusive. The process is linear—one problem, one set of symptoms, one cure. In Chinese theory this is not possible. Two people with colon cancer could be diagnosed quite differently. One person's system might be "damp," another's "dry." The phases and blockages could be opposite. Treatment points would be different in each case. To find enough people who need the exact points treated over the course of the disease is rare. To conduct Western-style studies with large test and control groups becomes complicated. It can be done, as discussed below; but to date, acupuncturists, like most Eastern (and in fact, Western) practitioners, use case histories and clinical practice as the basis for what works.

Studies do exist, despite the difficulties, in international and national medical journals, explaining in scientific terms the usefulness of acupuncture for a variety of ills from depression and pain to inflammation and paralysis. For example, Margaret Naeser, associate research professor of neurology at Boston University Medical School, uses acupuncture to treat paralysis in those who have suffered strokes. She first observed such treatment in China. Impressed by the improvements in strength and mobility, she came home to conduct her own research. Her study "compared real versus sham acupuncture in the treatment of paralysis in acute stroke patients, and examined the results in relationship to

CT scan lesion sites." Improvement was significant in the real acupuncture patients. There was no change in patients receiving sham acupuncture. Naeser is currently publishing information on these promising techniques.[47]

The benefits of Chinese medicine most widely recognized in the United States today, however, are in the areas of pain and anesthesia. The results here are more easily discernible. Whereas doctors in the 1970s, when acupuncture was first introduced here, claimed that the results were placebo effects (thinking it will work and thus it does), such attitudes over time and with observation are harder to maintain in the face of surgery. If you cut someone's abdomen open without anesthesia, you can count on their feeling it no matter what they're thinking. In China, acupuncture needles were used on specific points to block pain during surgery, with few or no drugs. Today acupuncture and small amounts of drugs are more likely to be combined.

Curious American teams have witnessed this, filmed it, and imported it. One journalist experienced it firsthand. James Reston of the *New York Times* some years ago needed emergency surgery for a ruptured appendix while in China. Imagine his surprise when he found that he was to receive acupuncture as part of the treatment for pain. His surprise changed to interest in a good story when he experienced the benefits firsthand.[48] Some skeptics still claim a placebo effect. But when the evidence of drug-free, painless surgery on dogs is presented, a skeptical posture is harder to sustain.

Thus, acupuncture to block pain, whether surgical or dental, headaches or cramps, is slowly finding acceptance, if not regular use, in mainstream medicine. Another use is in our continuous battle against drug and alcohol addiction. This is the use that most intrigues students in my classes. Terry Courtney, who launched the first detox acupuncture clinic in Boston in the late 1980s, learned of this approach from the Lincoln Hospital program in the South Bronx. This detox clinic, started in the 1970s, reports remarkable success rates with addicts. No one gets or expects 100 percent triumphs in this complex endeavor, but studies on acupuncture treatments are showing higher detox and lower recidivism than any other approach, including the dominant one of methadone. Other clinics have opened in the Boston area, as well as around the country.

Milton L. Bullock and colleagues conducted a placebo-controlled, single-blind study (the practitioners knew who were receiving specific points versus nonspecific, sham points; the participants did not) of eighty severe recidivist alcoholics. In the treatment group, twenty-one of the forty people finished the program with significant detoxification effects still present at the end of six months. In the control group (sham points) only one of the forty completed the program, with more than twice the number expressing a need for alcohol.[49]

Judge Stanley Goldstein, of Miami Beach, Florida, offers all first-offense drug offenders acupuncture detox treatment rather than jail. In the three years that he's made this offer, only 3 percent have been rearrested, compared with 33 percent in regular court. Length of treatment averages seventeen months. Goldstein reports: "What we've ended up with is nothing short of amazing." Other cities, too, have found it amazing. Portland, Oregon; Dayton, Ohio; and Oakland, California, have patterned drug courts on Judge Goldstein's model, and interest is growing.[50] In Portland, acupuncture is required before addicts can try methadone. Previously the first line of defense against addiction, methadone is now the last resort.[51]

When Terry Courtney comes to my classes, she brings pictures and videos explaining the treatment for an addict: once a day for forty-five minutes, five days a week for several weeks, followed by a varying schedule based on the individual's progress. As in all drug rehabilitation programs, counseling is recommended.

The treatment consists of five slim, short needles inserted in detoxification and relaxation points of each ear. One journalist, Nancy Waring, found the success rate, even with those who had "tried everything," impressive. One of her interviewees reports: "After years of failing at other things, I just wanted to give acupuncture a try."[52] Like many clients, this man, a crack addict, is more than pleased with the results, even though no one fully understands how it works. Waring notes:

Exactly how stimulating these points eases drug withdrawal and reduces cravings is not fully understood, but studies show that the release of endorphins, the body's own pain relieving, relaxation-inducing opiates is partly responsible. . . . [But] even those enthusiastic about acupuncture detox are aware that it may not be the best course of treatment for everyone. Skeptics, for their part, cite the lack of long-term studies. But with no sure cures and many more addicts than there are spaces in treatment programs, no one disputes that acupuncture detox is worth watching.[53]

And watched it is. Judge Goldstein is content with his short-term success rates. Others are accumulating statistics, watching the results with keen interest. In fact, it is through the back door of drug treatment that acupuncture may find its way into general health care, especially for chronic diseases, those diseases with which conventional medicine has the least success.

Anesthesia and drug detoxification speak a language of process and results graspable by Western doctors even if not fully understood. Using needles to block pain folds in with current research in medicine on blocking pain in general, whether through drugs or needles. Furthermore, to watch acupuncture accomplish this during surgery is impressive. Similarly, in detox the concentration is on endorphins, a hot medical topic, something the medical profession can understand.

A current theory is that heroin addicts lack endorphins and thus crave drugs to fill this void. Acupuncture, unlike methadone, revives the body's own ability to create endorphins, a natural high, decreasing the need for heroin. This is a concept medicine can work with. Unlike Chi or meridians, endorphins are familiar. Thus, it is through these two avenues that acupuncture is slowly working its way into medical and public imagination in the United States.

Perhaps it is stories like that of Tim Fortugno, a pitcher for the California Angels, that in the end will sway the public. In college, signed by the Oakland Athletics, Fortugno "blew out" his pitching arm. Nothing helped. Orthopedists, along with every known specialist, were sought, to no avail. His contract was canceled before he even began. A friend talked him into trying acupuncture. It worked. Today, in his thirties, his arm intact, he's pitching his best games. What could be more compelling than the return to form of a top athlete? Forget the drug addiction and chronic pain stories. Tim Fortugno may be all that's needed to mainstream acupuncture in North America.[54]

In England, more open to acupuncture, the popular view is different. In London a famous acupuncturist treats skin diseases. People line up around the block, waiting their turn for the unfixable to be fixed. Ask North Americans what acupuncture does best, and Tim Fortugno notwithstanding, they will probably answer, "Pain relief." Ask the English the same question, and they may be more likely to say, "Skin disease."

In fact, in both England and America acupuncturists treat a wide variety of health problems, from arthritis to cancer, from fatigue to the flu, from constipation to heartburn. Despite the wide applications to detox and pain prevention in the United States and skin diseases in the United Kingdom, the majority of an acupuncturist's work, like that of a conventional general practitioner or family practice physician, covers a broad range, from acute to chronic illnesses, mild to severe diseases.

Drew, like my students, was fascinated that a few needles in the ears could relax and detox long-term, hardened crack and heroin addicts. He was equally impressed with acupuncture used as anesthesia. But, he pointed out, he had a tumor; he wasn't a drug addict. He didn't feel well, but he wasn't in a lot of pain, and he knew he didn't want his head cut open without conventional anesthesia. So what did acupuncture have to offer him? These were excellent questions. The answers weren't so clear. Traditional acupuncturists would have responded that a tumor was a sign of major imbalance. Surgery, drugs, and radiation might alleviate the obvious problems but would stress his already out-of-whack body further. Do the surgery, have the radiation, but rely on other modalities to restore harmony, to strengthen the body, calm the mind.

Coming from a Western orientation, my explanations focused on acupuncture as a means to boost his immune system and release endorphins to give him a natural, calming high amid all of the frenzied lows he faced each day. He had talked with Val, my acupuncturist, and decided for himself. Probably I was pushier than I remember. In any case he had gone, at least to ask.

After his initial interview with Valerie, Drew was amenable. He liked her approach to his illness. He liked her open, supportive manner, and he liked her. Val worked with a physician in his office. Drew, making so many new adjustments, enjoyed at least some familiarity there—a doctor's office with the usual accoutrements.

In the first week home from his first surgery, I took my weak and bundled-up son to Val. Her approach was to work aggressively on strengthening him, physically and emotionally, so that his body could do the healing. She chose not to work on the cancer. She explained that in China a practitioner, when treating cancer with Chinese medicine, might see the patient five or six times a week. Accompanying the treatments would be extensive use of Chinese herbs. The process would be aggressive, sometimes painful, and time-consuming. It would be the primary force toward a cure. Just as Drew's life revolved around the hospital, his numerous doctors, and lab visits, an Eastern approach would have him equally busy with the Chinese methods. Since Western medicine was dominant here, she acted as supplementary care. Further, Val felt that if Drew were to take herbs, she would refer him to an herbal specialist. There are remarkable success stories for a variety of illnesses using herbal remedies, but Drew couldn't face another practitioner. He was doing enough.

Val treated the cancer indirectly by enhancing Drew's general health. From the beginning she said his pulses showed a strong constitution. Working from this base, she enhanced his chances of recovery by first treating his immune system. Her aim was to safeguard his system by working to block new cancer cells and keep him strong against other illnesses, such as the endless round of New England winter flus. Throughout the two surgeries and radiation she worked to counteract the invasiveness of these lifesaving but weakening procedures by keeping his metabolism steady and his energy flowing smoothly.

During the radiation she concentrated on detoxification from the radiation itself, as well as from the breakdown of cancerous cells. As the body rejects toxic waste, whether drugs or cells, the elimination process stresses the body and can mirror the symptoms of the illness itself. For example, removing the formaldehyde from my body gave me the same symptoms as when it went into my body. Such a process has to be done slowly and carefully so as not to overwhelm.

An extreme example of too rapid detoxification can be seen in bird migration. When birds feast on pesticide-poisoned grass or insects, the toxins store in their body fat and muscles. When they migrate south, they burn fat and exercise muscles, often resulting in death—literally falling from the sky—poisoned by toxins in their bodies being released too quickly. Thus, although detox in Drew's case was not life-threatening, Val worked to minimize the side effects of radiation by trying to release slowly the excess toxins before they could build up.

Val's approach was at the general level of immunity, strengthening, and detoxification. She also attended to the specific. On each visit she focused on points relevant to what Drew reported that day. He occasionally had hovering headaches and later, during the radiation, she intervened to stop nausea and fatigue when they were on the verge of happening. Drew also experienced hormonal fluctuations as varied supplemental levels were being tried to replicate his defunct pituitary gland. Hot flashes, fatigue, and other symptoms were corrected by regulating his hormone supplements, bolstered by on-the-spot acupuncture.

Another important, less tangible area of treatment was emotional help. Like Eastern practitioners in general, acupuncturists do not separate the mind from the body. The emphasis is on restoring a quality of life that encompasses a healthy body and a calm, strong mind. Thus, in acupuncture the practitioner-patient relationship is part of the cure. Val explained, "The quality of my interactions with patients is important. I try to establish a good relationship. I've never met an acupuncturist who wasn't interested in dealing with a patient as a person rather than a cluster of symptoms. It's intrinsic to the approach. I have to know what kind of mood someone is in, background about the person's family life and professional life to round out my assessment of them."

The psychoemotive level in a person is defined as the finer, subtler level on a continuum on which the physical is seen as the grosser, more obvious manifestation of a person's health. To understand a person's condition and to treat that condition, these different elements have to be considered. "Symptomatically, most of the time patients will have emotional tendencies consistent with physical disharmonies in our system of classification," Val noted.

In Drew's case, Val felt he was well adjusted on the psychoemotive level. His main problems were physically displayed. "He came to acupuncture very clear and ready to deal with his emotions around his health—different from many people who have emotional difficulty facing it all." Talking with Val helped Drew remain emotionally steady.

She offered support during each acupuncture visit. Drew could talk with her openly, and she was available to him both as a listener and as a practitioner. She worked with acupuncture to relax him. Part of every treatment was to generate a calm energy, an endorphin high, something he could feel immediately and keep with him to face the rest of his troubling life. It was this part that hooked Drew to acupuncture. He went two or three times a week, lay down on a comfortable examining table, and talked with Val about his symptoms, concerns, and fears. She placed the needles in the appropriate places and left him to relax for fifteen to twenty minutes. With soft classical background music, Drew went into a deep relaxation, often falling asleep.

Counseling and Cancer

Illness allows you to be self-centered, to put yourself first. Many become drenched with self-pity, an understandable but debilitating mood. While concentrating all of his energies on recovery, Drew never exhibited the understandable "why me?" attitude, with which we all would have sympathized. His focus was on getting well, not wallowing in being sick.

That didn't mean painful questions didn't reside just under the surface. Although Val felt his emotional health was good, Drew decided to see a counselor, a psychotherapist, to explore these fumblings. Better to deal with them now and learn from them than have to rediscover them, more deeply entrenched, years later. Once again, my university offered support through its counseling center. Drew went to a wonderful man, Paul, who encouraged him to indulge himself for this one hour a week in whatever he wanted to talk about. Drew didn't have to worry about distressing Paul with his fears. He could open the wounds and let them rip, with a less involved but gentle man to guide him, a man who cared a lot yet wasn't going to weep with him or feel his pain as searingly as he (or Stephen and I) did. This relationship lasted for six months. It started when radiation began and ended in May with the close of school. Drew found it a reprieve from the physical: We all felt he had handled having cancer too well. Counseling gave him an avenue to explore the seamier side of cancer, the weaknesses and the loathings. Drew also explored with Paul the effects his having cancer had on his relationships with others. He was, after all, deeply changed. Drew now, for example, faced renewing his relationship with Rebecca. Rebecca returned from China in December 1991, three days before radiation was to begin. (She had offered to come home before the first surgery. Drew talked her out of it.) Both had been through the most profound experiences of their lives; but those experiences were very different, and they went through them separately. Rebecca, age twenty, from a small, close-knit family in small-town and rural Vermont, had traveled around the world, geographically and metaphorically, to China. Drew had undergone two major surgeries for a malignant tumor bordering his brain. Neither could fully understand the vast dimensions of the other's changes. Drew had never been out of the Western world. Rebecca had never been seriously ill.

By the time Rebecca returned, Drew looked and felt quite well. His hair flopped over his scull scar. He was gaining weight and energy. He didn't look like a cancer patient. Rebecca, relieved to see him so well, presumed his illness was mostly over. Drew, in an emotional sense, had waited for Rebecca's return for it to really begin. His expectations were higher, more grandiose, than possibility allowed. All of those hours in MRI chambers holding onto Rebecca's image, all of the fantasies; nothing in real life could match those dreams. Paul helped Drew sort this out.

Drew and Rebecca held on. At age twenty-one and twenty, they did what many people of any age can't do in a crisis—they talked to each other and to friends, they wrote their thoughts and expectations down, they spent time apart, they came together. Rebecca could have walked away. She didn't. Drew could have withdrawn, claiming he had been through enough. He didn't. They struggled with the beast and beat it. Paul helped with this complicated journey.

Counseling and acupuncture combined with diet and relaxations to make Drew feel rested and calm, with renewed energy to face the struggles of getting well. He liked these strange new strategies. His friends and family loved hearing about them. Many wanted to try them.

Once again, everyone but the doctors was curious. But no doctor was against Drew's healing methods. Universally, their attitude was that if Drew wanted to do them, if he thought they helped—fine, then do them.

Drew wanted to do them, and he indeed did do them; he did them all. And just in case Norman Cousins and the *Reader's Digest* were right, that laughter is the best medicine, he watched hilarious movies, covering all bases.

Chapter Seven

ROBUST RESISTANCE

W ell, I guess this is it." Dr. R smiled on the last day of Drew's radiation treatment. I had come along on this momentous day to discuss long-range plans for follow-up. Dr. R was the doctor we had seen the most. Drew saw him regularly for over two months. I had come to the center occasionally. Dr. R was the only doctor we encountered who consistently had time to talk and to listen. In the beginning he had chatted with all of us. What did we do? Where did we come from? How were we coping? He gave us large chunks of his time, he was never rushed, he asked about Drew's life as well as his health, and he listened carefully. His research and practice limited him to a few carefully chosen patients. These lucky few got his full attention.

Although I didn't go with Drew for most of his radiation, when I did, Dr. R commented on how well Drew was doing physically and psychologically with the program. Certainly, compared to his fellow patients, Drew was a marvel of health.

Of all of the people Drew had worked with in the past months, Dr. R was the most open to different points of view and to being questioned.

He seemed the doctor most likely to be interested in the alternative methods Drew had experienced. Since the Japanese studies on radiation and diet seemed the most convincing and since Dr. R, a radiotherapist, might find them intriguing, Drew decided to start with these articles. He took me along, all of the studies at my fingertips. Dr. R and I had discussed our medical research interests at some length. Drew and I were optimistic that he could use some of what we had learned to help others cope with the myriad problems of radiation therapy.

Drew started explaining about how well he felt, connecting it to miso soup, seaweed, umeboshi plums. I, in my most academic voice, inserted scientific data, study after study. Drew had decided to start small—a few easily used, inexpensive remedies accessible to all.

Dr. R listened carefully, smiling at Drew's references to his initial reactions to seaweed. Dr. R was unfailingly polite. But the longer Drew talked, the less this expert communicator listened. Something had switched off. I told him I had all of the references if he was interested. He smiled his broad, sincere smile, looked Drew right in the eye and said, "Drew, the main thing is it made *you* feel better to do it. For that I'm happy. The main thing here is your great attitude."

In other words, do what works for you. You believe it, do it; it'll work. Placebo effect. Nothing generalizable here. Of course, Dr. R was right about Drew's attitude—it is great. But attitude is not enough. He'd always had a great attitude. That didn't stop his getting cancer. And how great would his outlook have remained if he'd had to live with piercing headaches or extreme nausea and fatigue? No, Dr. R was not interested. He was interested in Drew; he was genuinely happy that he was doing so well. He had no curiosity at all about alternative treatments, even those embedded in careful, suggestive research.

Lack of curiosity. It always surprises me, especially in such clever people. Ten years ago doctors were likely to try to dissuade, to dismiss as quackery, to rage against the absurdity of anything other than conventional medical treatment. That still happens occasionally but is far less common. No one objected to what Drew was doing. No doctor stormed into Drew's hospital room demanding that he eat the hospital's food. Doctors, nurses, and staff either thought it a good idea to avoid hospital cuisine or were indifferent to what he ate. No one treated Drew as deviant when he mentioned visualization or acupuncture. He was, in fact, consistently treated with respect. The attitude was "If it works for you, do it, but I don't need to know anything about it. This is your thing."

People writing about healing themselves report the same phenomenon. In the case of Kit Kitatani, the United Nations specialist, even doctors who encouraged him with his diet showed no curiosity about what exactly he was eating. "After realizing he was getting better, they told him to continue with what he was doing, but they didn't want to know more about it."[1]

Herb Walley, with prostate cancer in his early forties, had a similar experience. His doctor instructed him, " 'If the tests showed [*sic*] no cancer, then just keep on doing whatever you're doing.' He had no knowledge of, or desire to learn about, macrobiotics. All tests came back negative."[2]

Elaine Nussbaum's oncologist understood that she was more committed to macrobiotics than to conventional treatment. Perhaps because she was so riddled with cancers and, in the doctor's own words, her chances of recovery were "as close to zero as you can get," the doctor accepted her decision. The doctor still monitored Nussbaum's progress and shared in her joy and recovery.

"Here comes my miracle," my oncologist smiled at me when Ralph and I came into her office.

"I'm not surprised," I responded. "I knew what the results would be."

"I'm not surprised either," she admitted, and she showed me the initial report from the radiology department.

There was no cancer in my lungs or my bones.[3]

The doctor called her a miracle. She wasn't surprised that Nussbaum had overcome her zero chances and had not treated her as crazy for trying macrobiotics. She had been a one-doctor fan club. But once again, here was a doctor with access to what might have caused this "miracle," and she wasn't interested. No curiosity from an oncologist, someone who must face as many failures as successes on a daily basis. Had the doctor inquired into Nussbaum's harrowing journey from death's door to recovery, she might question the use of the word *miracle*. In fact, recovery was a result of struggle and hard work on Nussbaum's part and that of her family.

If so many doctors, when presented with evidence of potentially successful treatment plans in the face of such devastation from cancer, show no curiosity, then the salient questions are why, how come, how can this be.

Many medical watchers and writers focus on the roles of power, greed, and money in our health care system. Doctors cling to what they

know, excluding the new, in order to maintain control. The more out-
siders who emerge, the more control is required to keep them out. The
medical power base, expressed through the American Medical Association (AMA), is increasingly in jeopardy from such institutional factors as
rising costs and threats in the form of national health coverage and big-
business, for-profit hospital takeovers, as well as from growing public
dissatisfaction with current medical care. In response it tries to tighten
its hold and control the increasingly uncontrollable. A lot is at stake: self-
regulation, a free-market profession, and tremendous amounts of money
in the form of corporate profits (to pharmaceutical and insurance companies, for example) and physician incomes.

Corporate profits and industry-government overlaps have been explored in depth for years by consumer advocates like Ralph Nader and
scholars such as Paul Starr and Howard Waitzkin. Ralph Moss's 1989
book, *The Cancer Industry*, rekindles the flame of 1970s outrage about
how illness is managed in America. A couple of examples: (1) In the
1980s the CEO for the parent company of Hooker Chemical Company
(of Love Canal fame) was also the head of the President's Cancer Panel;
and (2) the board of overseers for Sloan-Kettering Cancer Center, the
largest private cancer center in the world, draws almost a third of its
members from the chemical, oil, and car industries, and another third
are leading financiers; other board members include drug company ex-
ecutives and, incredibly, tobacco industry barons. Government, industry, and cancer organizations seem to be inextricably connected. Is it any
wonder that genetic codes and individual life-styles are investigated to
the exclusion of environmental factors? Alternative medicines? Fewer
drugs needed? Cleaner food, air, and workplaces required? Forget it.
Too much money to be lost there. Better to concentrate on cellular
structures, it seems.

Individual doctors and medicine as a whole are described by one
writer as "pursu[ing] economic self-interest just like everyone else, and
arrangements that maximize income are always going to be looked upon
favorably by those whose incomes are maximized."[4] But the high costs
of maintaining that self-interest and our burdened medical system are
astronomical, and no one, including orthodox medicine, is happy about
it. In 1930, 3.5 percent of the American gross national product went to
health care; by 1990, 12.2 percent did. Everyone—doctors, hospitals, the
public—agrees change is necessary. The controversy arises only when it
comes to what the changes will look like, where to cut.

These economic critiques are relevant for what ails our health care system as well as what keeps medicine an empire. After all, only in the early 1990s did the United States administratively move toward a national health plan, the last industrialized country to do so.

Money and power are clearly parts of the problem. Yet shocking as some of the economic arguments are, they are not enough; such explanations don't account for behaviors of individual doctors. Dr. R was not thinking of money or power when his eyes glazed over after two minutes of alternative talk. Nussbaum's friendly, even supportive oncologist, welcoming her with a cheerful "Here comes my miracle," was not afraid macrobiotics would put her out of business. No, the problem goes deeper than money. Belief systems also play a crucial role. A friend recently gave her internist a copy of Sherry Rogers's book, *Tired or Toxic*, a book that looks at our current environment, how it causes disease, and what to do about it. Although conventionally trained, Rogers is by no means a conventional doctor. My friend's internist said he would read it; he didn't. He sent it back to her with a note explaining that if he read it he might have to completely change his orientation to health and illness, a change he couldn't face making.

People in general and institutions in particular are slow to change. We all hold onto what we know to make sense of our lives and worlds. And as worlds change ever faster, more chaotically, the more strongly we are apt to hold onto what we understand until we can incorporate changes into our knowledge base with the least disruption. Historically, this has been particularly true of medicine. The germ theory, the cornerstone of modern medicine, had as hard a time being accepted in the nineteenth century as holistic or alternative understandings do today. The very idea of bacteria, germs as microscopic organisms that could make people sick, was foreign to medical men. For example, in the mid-eighteenth century, two British obstetricians, Gordon of Aberdeen and White of Manchester, argued that childbed fever was contagious. They were ignored. One hundred years later, Oliver Wendell Holmes repeated their argument: "The disease known as puerperal fever is so far contagious as to be frequently carried from patient to patient by physicians and nurses."[5] Holmes offered a method of prevention, suggesting that obstetricians take care to separate postmortems from deliveries. He was not ignored but scorned: Hugh Hodge and Charles Meigs, leading American obstetricians of the day, ridiculed and "refuted" his work.[6]

In 1861, Ignaz Phillip Semmelweiss published *The Cause, Concept and Prevention of Childbed Fever*. Semmelweiss had noticed that childbed fever was less prevalent in hospitals when midwives instead of doctors delivered babies. Surmising that attendance at postmortems was the culprit, he initiated the practice of scrubbing up in chlorine water and using a nail brush before seeing a patient. The mortality rate from childbed fever dropped. Semmelweiss, however, was ostracized.[7]

Why did the germ theory generate such resistance? In part it challenged the status quo, the known, the illusion of certainty in one's belief system. The new approach was not yet well understood—unseeable germs, much like meridians, required a leap of faith. Knowledge of the role of bacteria and viruses was limited, and to suggest that cleanliness and health might be related probably seemed farfetched. As Thomas Kuhn has discussed, we have a long legacy of resistance to new ideas in science that require great bounds,[8] and the same can be seen in medicine. Furthermore, doctors are trained to be healers, not harmers. For them to reconceptualize the death of patients as iatrogenic (doctor-induced) was not an easy task. Whenever doctors feel challenged, the implication is that what they do is not enough. To question their brand of medicine is to question their ability to heal. It is only a short step to the slippery slope of questioning whether they are harming as well as healing. Many find it easier to dismiss the challenging and the challenger rather than face the shock of the new. In the case of germs, as has been true with modern challenges such as the changing role of nutrition in heart disease, resistance decreased as times changed and evidence piled up.

By the late 1870s, the work of Robert Koch and Louis Pasteur in the development of bacteriology had made it impossible to ignore further the role of germs in disease. Writing of antisepsis, Joseph Lister observed in 1867:

Previously to its introduction the two large wards in which most of my cases of accident and of operation are treated were among the unhealthiest in the whole surgical division of the Glasgow Royal Infirmary. . . . But since the antiseptic treatment has been brought into full operation, and wounds and abscesses no longer poison the atmosphere with putrid exhalations, my wards, though in other respects, under precisely the same circumstances as before, have completely changed their character; so that during the last nine months not a single instance of pyaemia, hospital gangrene, or erysipelas has occurred in them.[9]

The war on germs had begun.

The increasingly sophisticated discovery of microorganisms and methods of treatment in this century have led to massive campaigns against disease. After World War II, as these campaigns grew more successful, optimism for the end of disease abounded in the medical profession and the general public. And indeed, great strides in health care were made—polio vaccines, antibiotic cures, more recently the field of imaging (such as MRI), and so forth. Modern medicine, derived in part from chemical warfare, was applied to eradicate disease, and medical metaphors, in fact, became deeply militaristic: "the war on AIDS," "the eradication of the enemy," and the like. The body became (and remains) a battlefield, with good doctors fighting the good fight against bad bugs. The ill find themselves in a unique position. Perri Klass, in her book on her medical education, sums up this fight:

> If we are at war, then who is the enemy? Rightly the enemy is disease, and even if that is not your favorite metaphor, it is a rather common way to think of medicine: we are combatting these deadly processes for the bodies of our patients. They become battlefields, lying there passively in bed while the evil armies of pathology and the resplendent forces of modern medicine fight it out. . . . The real problem arises because all too often the patient comes to personify the disease, and somehow the patient becomes the enemy.[10]

In this war, the assumption is that all diseases can be conquered. First, the enemy is defined and then cordoned off. An active doctor and passive patient agree "the doctor knows best." Specific etiology (causation), with an emphasis on the cell or a particular organ rather than the whole person, is the focus. Even as some researchers start to expand the germ theory model with explorations of strengthening the body's immune system as a means to create balance and thus health, the battlefield image remains intact. One team of researchers writing on, what else, the "war on cancer," addresses the "immune surveillance system." Instead of doctors playing gunmen attacking outlaws—germs—these writers suggest the need to stimulate the body's own "defensive system by which immune cells patrol silently throughout the body, attacking foreign invaders."[11] Activate those "killer cells." In this newer landscape of the body, a continuous defend-and-conquer scenario unfolds in each of us, sick or well, all of the time. Reflections of military strategies against disease show up in literature as well as medical discussion. In Jeanette Winterson's *Written on the Body*, the narrator mourns a lover's diagnosis of chronic lymphocytic leukemia,

> In the secret places of her thymus gland Louise is making too much of herself. Her faithful biology depends on regulation but the white T-cells have turned bandit. They don't obey the rules. They are swarming into the

bloodstream, overturning the quiet order of spleen and intestine. . . . It used to be their job to keep her body safe from enemies on the outside. They were her immunity, her certainty against infection. Now they are the enemies on the inside. The security forces have rebelled. Louise is the victim of a coup.[12]

Despite many advances in medicine using such war-based metaphors, optimism that aggressive, scientific medicine can eradicate or cure all diseases has diminished by the late twentieth century.

Repeatedly, polls show public dissatisfaction with health care in the United States; the costs are too high, doctors don't listen, and so forth. At the same time, the public, each day, places inordinate trust in this system. And the breakthroughs such as imaging, proton beam radiation, and laser surgeries *are* stunning. Doctors find themselves in a paradoxical situation: On the one hand, they face enough failure and criticism to make them defensive (and in need of enormous amounts of malpractice insurance); on the other, they experience enough success and devotion to promote arrogance. Neither posture is conducive to change or openness to new paradigms. Alternative models of health care, while perhaps complementary with orthodox medicine, may be only perceivable as threats, based on their differences, their otherness, from the safety of the known, even if the known changes daily. Certainly, the alternatives I've discussed in this book *are* different. From their conceptual roots to actual practice they are as *other* to Western medical thought as possible. For example:

• Where Western medicine looks for the single cause, Eastern medicine assumes multiple ones.

• Where Western medicine's focus is on curing illness, Eastern medicine attempts to prevent it. When Western medicine does go for prevention, the approach is still quintessentially Western. For example, a controversial experiment is underway whereby healthy women at high risk of developing breast cancer are to be given a drug—an antiestrogen, tamoxifen—to see if it prevents the disease. Rita Arditti, a sociologist specializing in women and cancer, writes about this experiment's critics: "The criticisms center around the fact that tamoxifen causes liver cancer in rats, liver changes in all species tested, and that a number of endometrial cancers have been reported among tamoxifen users."[13] Do healthy women already at higher than average risk for breast cancer need to add possible liver or endometrial cancer to their fears? If the West is going to shift to a prevention model, it will have to do better than this.

• Where Western medicine defines knowledge hierarchically, with the doctor the knower and the patient the known—the former active, the latter passive—Eastern medicine centers on a partnership of knowers. In this partnership each has a different kind of knowledge, and all of the players are active participants. Patients become people responsible for making decisions about their treatment and recovery. Experts offer guidance and information, treatments and support, but ill people decide what they are willing or able to do to ease their situation. This is not a blame-the-victim message of total responsibility but rather a means to feel in power, in control of one's own life decisions instead of being a helpless victim of disease processes and the experts that tend to them.

This Western inequality between doctor and patient is powerfully summed up in Alan Bennett's play about the medical miseries of and ministrations to King George III. In a stark scene, King George sits pitifully strapped into a chair, barefoot and disheveled, clothed in a tattered, stained nightdress, having been leeched, burned, purged, and pierced. He musters a shred of strength to proclaim to one of his overbearing physicians: "King: (Howling) 'I am the King of England.'"

His doctor, grandly dressed, elegantly erect, booms with authority to King George and to the audience: "No, sir. You are the patient."[14]

• Where Western medicine does battle against the enemies of disease with big guns, Eastern medicine seeks peace through balance. Disease, rather than being an invader, is a messenger from the body, signaling for help, change, and harmony. Elizabeth Kubler-Ross, well known to many for her help in coping with dying, says, "If one is in pain, comfort must be sought. The body is asking for something. Don't keep denying it."[15]

Vivien Newbold, talking about her own shifts in perspective as a Western doctor incorporating some Eastern values, tells a story of her experience with a lump in her breast.

Was this lump going to turn out to be a cancer to pay me back for all my bad habits? After obtaining a mammogram which indicated that the possibility of cancer was very remote and seeking macrobiotic counseling, I went on a strict diet. The lump disappeared; however, whenever I overindulged in rich food, the lump would reappear and be very painful. For the first few months, I was angry and resentful. I could not overindulge in the foods I enjoyed so much without a rude reminder from this wretched little thing. Then, one day, I woke up and realized how precious that little lump was. It was my warning light which signalled that I was really harming myself.[16]

Newbold went from fear to anger to gratitude. We are all familiar with the fear—fear of cancer, fear of pain, fear of death; and the anger—anger at our bodies for betraying us, anger at something or someone for letting such terrible things befall us. The idea of gratitude where illness is concerned is indeed a stretch for the imagination. But it is all more complicated than I used to think. I'm not grateful, per se, that I developed environmental sensitivities, but I'm glad that what I learned from that experience helped Drew. None of us is grateful that Drew got cancer. In fact, we are still coping with the fear and the anger—a fear and anger that are appropriate and probably will never fully disappear. But Drew had no control over developing a tumor. He only had choices to make once he knew he had it. So why not, along with all of the enormous variety of emotions, treasure some of the close moments, delight in the new sense of one's own courage? The importance of every moment is fresh in Drew's mind regardless of how long or short his life may be. No one, no disease can take this away from him. He has been given a terrible gift. The Chinese philosophy that holds that buried in the seeds of danger are the seeds of opportunity helps to steady the nerves and build strength out of the ashes of weakness.

• Where Western medicine seeks proof and tangible evidence, striving for a practice based on experiments, validity, and controlled studies, Eastern medicine looks to clinical and historical experience, empirical knowledge passed down for thousands of years.

• Where the West looks to parts of the body, the individual organ or cell, utilizing skills that zero in on the part, separating the mind from the body, the East expands to the entire person, both body and mind considered part of the whole organism. In an obviously extreme but telling example in Western medicine of the part becoming more important than the whole (taken from an "AIDS Quarterly" segment on PBS television), one doctor advocated continuing an experimental AIDS drug despite the patient's worsening condition on the medication. His reason: the blood work showed improvement. Luckily for the ill man, the principal investigator (P.I.) of the experiment discontinued the drug. In an argument with his colleague, the P.I. pointed out that the blood work didn't matter; the patient was dying. The junior doctor reluctantly agreed to stop the experiment on this person and on others. But he wasn't convinced. After all, as he kept repeating, the blood work looked good.

Such an approach, in which a test result can become more important than the empirical evidence and a part of the body can be weighted over the person's well-being, would be unusual in an Eastern orientation to health and illness. Here the person is connected to the larger environment in a series of expansions and contractions, a push and pull relationship between matter and energy. Deep in its theoretical roots, modern Western physics is similar to the Eastern philosophy of expansion and contraction, yin and yang. The very structure of the atom is based on attraction and repulsion, an ongoing interplay of opposition and integration. Modern medicine, however, is not based on current physics, with its emphases from Werner Heisenberg and Albert Einstein on uncertainty and relativity. Rather it is embedded in the more graspable, concrete biological sciences.

Anthony Sattilaro, grappling with the differences between (1) his own training as a scientific physician and experiences as a patient in the Western mind's eye and (2) his introduction to and healing from the Eastern perspective, found himself challenging and changing his own assumptions.

I went from focusing my attention on viruses and cells under a microscope to sitting back and contemplating the vast interwoven mosaic of the universe. For example, when my back pain had returned, . . . I immediately believed the cancer had reawakened along my spinal column. The macrobiotic view was quite different. . . . According to [Eastern theory], the origin of my back pain was stagnation in a meridian that ran along my back, preventing energy . . . earth from freely passing along this meridian and nourishing my body. The two points of view are good examples of Western and Eastern thinking. The former addresses the effects, while the latter attempted to understand the correct causes. Once I accepted the Eastern view as possible, I began to gain a new appreciation of the vast interconnectedness of the universe.[17]

Sattilaro was indeed grateful for his expanded view of health and healing; "In treating my own cancer, I put this holistic view to the ultimate test and it saved my life."[18]*

Aesthetically and logically, Eastern methods of health and healing appeal to me more than the take-charge Western model does. The idea

---

*Unfortunately for Dr. Sattilaro, his life was saved only temporarily. Once cleared of cancer, he resumed his previous life-style. When he was well, he found that his dietary changes were difficult. He died of cancer some years later. Perhaps he would have had a recurrence anyway. This is impossible to know. In any case he lived longer than he or his doctors expected him to, and he credited this to his use of alternative methods.

of a holistic approach to treatment, the shift from passive patient to active participant, the ideal of prevention, all make sense to me. I prefer a movement toward a preventive, socially and environmentally aware model of health promotion rather than our current medical model of waiting for disease. But no one would argue that Eastern medicine saved Drew's life. In fact, Western medicine did. Heroic medicine, doing what it does best, isolating the affected area and attacking it, rode into town and indeed was heroic. Careful, scientific studies of bodily parts and technical fixes over the past decade radically improved the surgical techniques and radiation used. Without these innovations Drew's chances of survival were slim. Western medicine was crucial. Eastern medicines played a less obvious role. The help derived from such modalities as acupuncture were important but secondary.

One of my purposes in this book, however, is to integrate different understandings of medicine. Rather than an either/or approach, why not seek a blended model of medicine that allows for varied mixtures of treatments, depending on the problem. Just as Eastern medicine assumes a holistic view of the person, why not integrate the best of East and West to develop a holistic medical model working to improve people's health and thus their lives? In this book I've concentrated on the Eastern measures taken rather than the Western remedies because the Eastern approach is more ignored, less available to the American public despite growing awareness.

Drew benefited from the best of both. He used Eastern methods to be a more active patient in the Western model. He energetically set a course toward health that served him well. Acupuncture was used to stimulate his immune system, help diffuse his stress, and thus contribute to his physical and mental well-being. By daily visualizing the tumor's being replaced by healthy, glowing cells, he was reclaiming his body, making both the unhealthy and healthy cells a part of himself that he could navigate, instead of suffering rage at his own body. Rather than feeling betrayed, he could offer himself sympathy and constructive action. By eating foods that made him feel stronger during all of the curing but taxing events—surgeries, radiation, hospital procedures—he could feel an active partner in the process rather than a passive pawn. His rapid recoveries can be credited in part to these strengthening activities.

By feeling better, he could better tolerate the medical procedures and appreciate how much all of these processes were helping him. Radiation may be saving your life, but if you are too ill to eat or your head is pounding, it doesn't feel that way. Better to feel good while you're getting well. Drew believed he was working with the doctors to make himself well.

Here perhaps we can find some overlap between East and West. Both agree that attitude, while by no means the decisive element some would have us believe, is important to quality of life during the illness and important to getting over the illness. Judith Glassman, in her study of terminal cancer survivors, found that "[t]he most striking thing about all of these people is that each engineered his or her own recovery and each had an enormous will to live."[19] A feeling of control and participation in health care, so integral to Eastern medicine, is slowly inching its way into some Western practices.

In a review of thirty-four controlled studies, researchers found that when surgical or coronary patients were given information, support, or both to help them get through medical procedures, they did better than patients who received routine care. Hospital stays were reduced, and recovery time was decreased.[20] Similar results on information giving, mainly from the psychology and nursing literatures, have been shown in childbirth,[21] in difficult or painful physical exams,[22] and when the patient is a child.[23]

When Drew first entered the hospital, a nurse came to his room, did the usual vital-signs routine, and then whipped out a questionnaire. She explained that they had recently started asking how much people wanted to know. Did Drew want to be informed about the procedures? How detailed did he want the discussion to be? And so forth. She explained that some patients want to know nothing: "Just do what you have to do and get me out of here." Others want a sketchy picture but not too detailed. Still others want the full score; they want to know everything. Drew wanted the full score. She gave it to him, at least a technical one. She put his request in his file, and it seemed that every time we turned around, at least before the first surgery, he got it again. Frightening as it was, Drew found that knowing what to expect was easier than facing what his imagination could do with the unknown. There were already enough unknowns.

Increased patient control and participation lead to better understanding of the problem and the necessary treatment, which then come full circle to deliver more patient control. Rather than telling the ill to shape up, improve their attitudes, and assume total individual responsibility, research suggests that medical forces can help people develop the strength to face procedures by encouraging feelings of control.

Informing and thus activating ill people and utilizing alternative programs are recent developments in this country, incorporated by some, rejected by others. Despite ongoing changes, however, there are concrete and subtle obstacles to fundamental change within the medical community. An interpretation of modern scientific views within medicine offer perhaps one last note for understanding the whys of these obstacles. As discussed earlier, doctors want studies. They want proof. They want certainty. Sounds good. I do too. Wherever possible in this book, I too have relied on studies to make my points clearer and to make sense of the choices I've made about my health and helped Drew to make about his. As a sociologist, like doctors, I am more comfortable making decisions from a firm grounding.

The scientific method is rooted in a vision of pure, objective inquiry in which observed facts confirm or deny hypotheses. Once a hypothesis is tested repeatedly and confirmed, it becomes a law, a workable fact. Controlled studies in medicine require one group to be tested with the new procedure, test, or drug; the other group, not. If it is the preferred double-blind study, no one knows which group any patient is in. The mind is banished from the activities. Sounds good again: neat, clean, compact, a method that delivers truth. And sometimes it does. Much of medical progress in the form of dazzling technology is a result of this method—careful studies, whether blind or not. Proton beam radiation, primarily zapping the tumor instead of the healthy tissue, owes its origins to medicine marching ahead. Just a decade ago these techniques were not as refined for chondrosarcomas, the outcome more a danger than an opportunity.

Some scientists, however, like Stephen Jay Gould, are questioning too rigid, too concrete a perception of science: "I believe that science must be understood as a social phenomenon, a gutsy human enterprise, not the work of robots programmed to collect pure information."[24] Just because no one has yet thought of the hypothesis or tested its validity doesn't mean something doesn't exist or isn't useful. Just because questions haven't been asked doesn't mean there are no answers. What I interpret Gould calling for is more imagination, to use science as a means to broaden the landscape, not narrow it. If scientists were more sensitive to the multifaceted aspects of life, the uncertainties as well as the absolutes, different questions could be asked and methods developed to study medicines such as acupuncture.

Furthermore, as already pointed out, medical practice is based at least as much on clinical experience as on scientific inquiry. Despite this reality, doctors' responses to unknown areas are often to assume they don't exist. The problem (such as environmental illness) or the treatment (macrobiotics or acupuncture) can be dismissed. "Where are the studies?" "Where is the proof?" These may be appropriate questions, but if the studies haven't been done and the proof doesn't exist, then the rational response to questions about unknowns is "I don't know" or "I'd like to know more." In fact, scientific inquiry, by its own internal logic, focuses on asking questions, knowing that the answers shift like grains of sand. Modern medical thought all too often dismisses the unknowns, clings to the known answers, forgetting about the questions. To focus on the answers at the expense of the questions invites a rigidity that short-circuits the very knowledge medical science seeks. Thus, science, narrowly defined, can become a cloak behind which established health care hides, as well as a pathfinder with innovative research. A scientific cosmology can serve as a blinder. And it is exactly behind this cloak, these blinders, that many doctors remain when it comes to the unknown, in this case complementary treatments for cancer.

But not all doctors adhere to this strict a code. It is through the work of mavericks that we see the other side of a scientific worldview, a side that enlightens and encourages new visions. People, including scientists, may cling to the known, but the scientific enterprise in its deepest philosophical roots assumes change. In fact, the scientific revolutions of the sixteenth and seventeenth centuries opened doors to critical, rational inquiry—even of science itself. An open, excited mind, always looking for new, unexplored questions, should be integral to any scientific enterprise, even if that means changing the form of the inquiry as well as the content.

Thus, it is no surprise that some doctors, trained in scientific medicine, are at the forefront of pushing the borders of the medical model, expanding horizons. It is, after all, doctors trained in conventional medicine who have written the majority of books on visualization and meditation methods for healing. Environmental medicine is a new discipline—physicians interested in expanding medicine out from the cell to the environment, drawing on a variety of holistic understandings to do so.

Although not recognized by the AMA as a specialty, interest in environmental illness is slowly showing up in mainstream medicine. Massachusetts General Hospital, often ahead of its time, has opened a new group practice to treat "sick building syndrome," focusing on how materials in our environment can make us ill. The practice emphasizes diagnosis and treatment, and prevention and education as well. Acupuncture, still foreign to many if my students are indicators, was brought to this country by American doctors who had visited China, and it is increasingly being studied in hospitals here for a variety of diseases, as well as for pain and substance detoxification. And macrobiotics, still considered the most obscure of these methods, is drawing a small but interested following in medical circles.

When I asked a holistic doctor in California why he had incorporated alternative methods into his practice, he responded, "I began to feel that all I did was push pills. I wasn't making enough people feel better; I was often making them sicker. It was a gradual change for me from cure to prevention, from invasive procedures to gentler measures. I still prescribe drugs when necessary. I haven't abandoned my training. I've just added to it."

This doctor, like most alternative physicians, didn't start out suggesting macrobiotics or homeopathic remedies. Most started like Guillermo Asis, presently practicing in Massachusetts. "I went from conversations with my father, while a medical student in Argentina, about how people practicing alternative healing methods were a bunch of quacks to the time of my training in New Orleans, when I often wondered how much good or harm we were really doing to our patients."[25] Marc Van Cauwenberghe has a similar story: "There are no sicknesses, only sick people. I started to realize this in medical school, but then went right along studying diseases only and seeing people as 'cases.'"[26]

Guillermo Asis learned about macrobiotics in trying to help his best friend overcome pancreatic cancer. His friend wasn't interested, but Asis was. His practice today includes multiple practitioners in Eastern and Western techniques, with diet a central factor in his own life as well as in his care of others. In a secondhand bookstore, Marc Van Cauwenberghe came across a book on Eastern medicine and cancer by George Ohsawa. He too became intrigued. He sought out Michio Kushi and today, dividing his time between Virginia and Massachusetts, is a prominent counselor and lecturer on macrobiotics. As a physician, he believes that helping people by means of diet is the most important thing he can do for their health.

David Williams gave up one of the largest medical practices in Texas to edit a widely circulated newsletter called *Alternatives*. He and his editorial staff search the medical and alternative literatures worldwide, as well as collecting people's experiences, to produce a comprehensive publication accessible to all. Doctors read it (20% to 25% of subscribers), but it is written so that the general public can understand and use the information.

The stories go on and on, testimony to the frustration some doctors feel, confined within Western scientific training. The majority of those who made changes shifted slowly, including alternative modalities without losing sight of the benefits of their earlier training.

Another group of doctors took an alternative route, through their own ill health rather than that of their clientele. In my own research I have talked with physicians who have been ill themselves: surgeons needing surgery, gynecologists experiencing difficult births. It can be a sobering ordeal for a doctor to face another doctor, often a stranger, from that far side of the room where the sick live. They are shocked at how helpless they feel, how indifferent the doctor often is, how little information they receive even when they put their questions in doctor-talk. One surgeon who underwent a traumatic surgery told me, disbelief still in his voice two years later, "I'm a surgeon and he treated me this way. I couldn't believe it. I hate to think how he treats the guy off the street." Did this experience change how he treats patients? "Oh yes," he assured me. "Yes indeed. For one thing, I'll never again tell a patient 'You'll be jogging in two days.'"

Recently I visited Drew's grandfather in Washington, D.C. A retired physician and loyal AMA member for sixty-some years, he was in the hospital following a harrowing surgery with multiple complications. I asked, "Do you like your doctors?"

"They saved my life," he responded quickly.

"Yes," I agreed. "So you would kiss their feet and you love them. But do you like them? Are you pleased with how they treat you?"

"I don't know," he replied with a tired laugh. "I've never seen one of them for more than sixty seconds. Doctors don't have time for people any more. It's a serious problem."

The movie *Doctor* and the book *Heartsounds* strikingly portray similar experiences when doctors find themselves on the other side of the imaging screen. Some become more sympathetic doctors; others seek new definitions of health and how to achieve it.

Henry Altenberg, a physician, was diagnosed with a tumor that seemed to be both cancer and not cancer—talk about uncertainty. He had it removed from his thyroid and decided he needed to get healthier fast. He went to a health food store on a vague search, not knowing exactly what he was after. He talked with people, read books, found his way to the Kushis, and started macrobiotics. Aside from feeling better, he lost unwanted weight, and his cholesterol went down. Today he and his wife, Jean, a nurse, run a holistic health center in Maine.

Both Drew and I experienced unexpected health bonuses like these—side effects for once beneficial. Drew, always slightly snuffly, with postnasal drip a part of his normal life, discovered what it felt like to have a clear head. He was so used to sniffling, it hadn't occurred to him that it was possible not to sniffle. My list is longer. My cholesterol, high in my family, went down from 200 to 160. A light fungus behind my ears, a decade-old condition controlled only with cortisone cream, disappeared. My skin, always dry, became softer, smoother. Friends told me my face had a glow, which surprised them given my life for the past two years. Sinking deeper into the personal, I discovered that body odor and the need for deodorants are caused by eating animal products. Bill Walton, playing pro basketball for the Portland Trail Blazers in the 1970s, found that when he was a vegetarian the locker room odor, indifferently noticed before, now overwhelmed him.

Henry Altenberg was so impressed by the changes in his health and that of others that he started introducing macrobiotics into his practice, which specialized in family and child psychiatry: "I am prepared to share my knowledge and experience with those patients I encounter in my practice who wish to learn about macrobiotics. I am giving consideration to preparing more fully for this by taking formal training, in order to utilize it within my practice."[27]

Helen Farrell, specializing in the treatment of women with premenstrual syndrome (PMS), is another doctor who helped herself as well as her practice. In fact, it was a woman with PMS who introduced her to macrobiotics. PMS can include such disturbances as digestive and stomach troubles, reproductive problems, migraine headaches and sinus flareups, mood swings, insomnia, and a lack of concentration. Effective treatment, often elusive, needs to be varied and flexible. Farrell finds diet, individually tailored, and exercise key ingredients for relieving these symptoms. She has come to believe that PMS is not really PMS but rather "a collection or focus of symptoms that occur in the female body as a result of stress, especially nutritional stress" that becomes entwined with hormonal activity. Through diet she has relieved her own migraine headaches and her father's chronic nasal congestion by persuading him to give up dairy products. She offers patients guidelines for achieving the same relief. She admits "it is very difficult to introduce the average North American to macrobiotic cooking." However, she encourages them to go slowly, to include "fun food" so that they won't feel deprived as they ease into the changes. As people start to feel better, the diet becomes easier.[28]

People make changes in their lives for a variety of reasons. Terry Shintani became interested in macrobiotics when he discovered that vegetarians need less sleep. He learned that he could feel rested on five to six hours of sleep after only a few weeks on the diet. (Perhaps that is how he earned medical and law degrees as well as a master's in public health). Curiosity about food and sleep connections led him to look for research on the subject. He found scientific backing for his experiences: a diet low in fat and high in complex carbohydrates can improve REM (rapid eye movement) sleep.[29] I too sleep less, more deeply, and more restfully with the changes in my diet.

All of these doctors, whether discovering macrobiotics and other alternative approaches to illness for themselves or for their medical practices, incorporated what they found into their Western medical background rather than replacing that whole background. In fact, they and others argue that the different models are compatible and enhance rather than compete with each other.

Eastern practices can soften the harsh edges of the technologies so often needed to help cure—in Drew's case MRIs, blood tests, X rays, surgeries, radiation. For these treatments can be distancing and painful, making ill people feel alienated from their own bodies as well as their illness. Anatole Broyard, writer and former editor of the *New York Times Book Review*, sums this up eloquently, remarking that "since technology deprives me of the intimacy of my illness, it makes it not mine but something that belongs to science. I wish my doctor could somehow repersonalize it for me. It would be more satisfying to me, it would allow me to feel that I *owned* my illness."[30] Broyard wants more from his doctors; he wants help to reconnect himself to his body once the machines and bureaucracies have done their work. "Just as he orders blood tests and bone scans of my body, I'd like my doctor to scan *me*, to grope for my spirit as well as my prostate. Without some such recognition, I am nothing but my illness."[31] Broyard doesn't require that his doctors love him or wallow in his miseries. He just wishes his doctors would "*brood* on my situation for perhaps five minutes." But his doctor wouldn't brood on his illness, nor would the doctor "survey [his] soul as well as [his] flesh." Anatole Broyard reports that his doctors groped only for his prostate.

I used to think it was possible to change doctor-patient relationships, educating doctors to probe deeper than the prostate, the brain, the womb. And maybe it is. Rita Charon, a physician at Columbia Medical School, requires students in her classes to write narratives in their patients' voices to get closer to what the patient, the ill person, the other, experiences.[32] But her excellent teaching techniques were not in time for Anatole Broyard, who died medically unrequited in 1990.

Neither were her ideas in time for Drew, at least not this time around. He did indeed have excellent medical care, with occasional "groping for his soul" by some doctors. Even the great surgeon fleetingly reached out to him, tentatively but with tenderness. The antidote, however, for the alienation of all of the high tech, all of the tests, even those endless arm punctures when there seemed to be no more veins to tap, resided for Drew in the alternatives. He had to do the equivalent of switching computer programs in midstream. Meditations, visualizations, relaxation breathing techniques, seeing the inside of his head with his mind's eye, and later counseling, all retrieved him and his illness in one piece from the MRI chamber, the piercing radiating beam, and all of those tubes and gadgets. In fact, he could incorporate the curative powers of these technologies into his imagination, making them less alienating, more healing. Relaxation techniques soothed his soul as well as his body. He had Val, not a doctor but a practitioner, someone to "brood" on his illness with him on a regular basis. Everything mingled in his body and his mind to make him feel in the center of this full catastrophe rather than peripheral to it.

David Dodson brings all of the above together in his medical practice. He believes that just as yin and yang complement each other through diversity, so too do Western and Eastern medicines. "This [yin and yang] symbolizes my experience as a medical scientist: the more I learn scientifically about medicine and nutrition, the more beauty and power of macrobiotics to promote health becomes apparent to me. Thus science has no conflict [here]."[33]

Terry Shintani also finds the two complementary. Despite surprise from both camps that he so successfully combines the two in his life and medical practice, he sees alternative medicines and modern science "as two ways of looking at the same truth. One from the large 'macro' view, a more holistic but less precise view, and the other from a 'micro' view, a more precise analytical view but a somewhat narrower perspective."[34]

If only the many practitioners working in these areas would recognize each other. It would have been wonderful, for example, if Val and Dr. T had discussed what each was doing to help Drew, had made joint adjustments, whether in physical or psychosocial care, to enhance each other and thus maximize their efforts.

This doesn't mean each would have to become an expert in the other's work. After all, Dr. T works in surgery with and trusts anesthesiologists each day without being able to do what they do. Imagine that Dr. R's staff included a nutritionist learned in foods and vitamins to ease the radiation process—perhaps serving soothing bancha tea and vegetable dip or miso broth and rice balls in the waiting room rather than cake and coffee. People might leave with more spring in their step, the spring they were surprised that Drew had and were sorry they lacked. Such rapport and mutual acceptance would broaden public imagination of what health care can be. Such mainstreaming of alternative medicines would make them more accessible to people of all classes and more likely to be covered by insurance companies and government programs.

In fact, East and West are getting closer, at least in theory if not yet in practice, despite their many differences. Dietary recommendations of the heart and cancer associations, along with various government agencies, are basically what macrobiotic experts have been advocating for years. The power of the mind to contribute to illness, long acknowledged by modern medicine (perhaps overly so), is increasingly recognized as a power that can also heal. Instead of banishing the mind from healing in double-blind, placebo-effect studies, some are trying to cultivate this energy in beneficial ways. A recent *Time* magazine cover story on alternatives described acupuncture as on the verge of becoming a mainstream approach to illness. And the National Institutes of Health have recently allocated funds for a grand-scale study into alternative methods to better understand how they work and where they help the most. After all, macrobiotics literally means "long life," and who can argue with that?

Not Drew. He walked down two parallel roads: first, the Western way of surgeons, drugs, blood tests, MRIs, and radiation—the world of the body; second, the Eastern path of macrobiotics, meditations, acupuncture—the world of the body drenched in the mind. At the level of theory and practitioners the roads never met. At the level of experience they became integrally entwined in Drew's body, his life, and his recovery. East and West meshed, enhancing each other, offering Drew unique ways of healing and coping. He cultivated calmness and strength from eating a balanced diet, doing visualizations, going to acupuncture. Counseling gave him a sense of sureness about himself, increased his self-knowledge and introduced yet another learning experience. Surgery and radiation saved his life, giving him a profound appreciation for sophisticated technology and acute medical care.

In the end so many modalities came together, turning a dreadful time into a productive one. Drew learned more than he thought possible, at times more than he ever wanted to know. There are so many experiences, so many feelings, so much new information to sort out. Although at times perplexed that his life was ever so at risk, Drew's grateful he's alive to ponder the matter. And ponder the matter he does, when he's not too busy savoring every moment, taking all and nothing for granted.

CONCLUSION

Somehow I keep coming back to that jigsaw puzzle—the pure joy of it. I must have conveyed this to friends because we got six puzzles for Christmas. But its time had come and gone by then. All of the puzzles sit neatly stacked in the basement awaiting a visiting child or sick relative. It was just a moment, a flash of time, when a puzzle became a distraction, a shared activity, a salvation of sorts. A surreal time, really. Did we actually go through all of that? Was this healthy young man, now so energetic, so full of life, ever so sick? Or was it all just a terrifying hallucination? As I watch him take off for a summer of travel—no sitting in front of a computer screen all day this summer—it's hard to believe the sun hasn't always been warm, the breeze cool, my son well.

As summer comes, we all feel more settled. Drew finished his two courses. He won a math award in calculus. I tease him—the surgeries didn't damage his brain; they improved it. With the end of school, feeling fine, he put himself back into the world of the well, the world of the normal, the world of the young. Given our backgrounds, ages, and health histories, we have, quite naturally, chosen different paths.

The macrobiotic diet, such an integral part of my life, remains my preferred way of eating even in health. I love the food, and even more I love the way I feel when I eat this food. Surprisingly, when you change your diet, you change your life. People who write about these changes report greater clarity and calmness. They feel calmer but stronger. They work less and accomplish more. They feel better about themselves, others, their lives. I agree. It's seductive.

Drew, however, glad that he learned what he did, was eager to modify his life, to eat with friends in exotic restaurants or not think about food at all. He stopped routine relaxation exercises. He said goodbye to Val and acupuncture. But he holds onto the knowledge he gained. He avoids dairy products, which make him too congested. A clear head appeals to him. He eats fewer sweets and red meats. He eats more vegetables, beans, and whole grains when available. Perhaps he will avoid the high cholesterol that is a legacy from both my family and his father's. He knows he can use relaxation exercises in times of stress. He respects acupuncture should he be ill again. He's left all of this behind, to resume a more carefree life, but not so far behind that he can't grasp it if he needs it or help friends if they do. And having learned to communicate well with doctors, even great surgeons, and to navigate hospitals and the world of high tech, he's also happy to put these skills away for now.

On the one hand, Drew craves the end of illness and all of the attendant medical ministrations; but on the other, he wants to hold onto the intensity that came with it—the intoxication of his illness, as Anatole Broyard called it. Or as Vietnam War novelist Tim O'Brien writes, "It's a hard thing to explain to someone who hasn't felt it, but the presence of death and danger has a way of bringing you fully awake. It makes things vivid. When you're afraid, really afraid, you see things you never saw before, you pay attention to the world. . . . You become part of a tribe."[1]

Every moment buzzes, every second is tangible—that terrible gift again. Does such passion require crisis? Maybe, at least in the high voltage range. But each moment is still precious, more quietly so perhaps, but precious.

So the ending seems happy. Or is it the beginning? Are we putting cancer behind us, or will it always be in front of us? Probably both, for we are all quite different now. Life looks more fragile as we sift through these experiences. It's as though we walked out of a cave into a new consciousness, full of never-to-be-forgotten truths and fears, a new co-terie of dangers and opportunities—a new set of priorities that Drew strives to understand.

"Keep your eye on the ball," Drew said with a wry smile and a casual wave as he took off for the West. "Keep your eye on the ball."

EPILOGUE BY DREW TODD

As a child, I never went to camp. It wasn't until the summer of 1993, one week after graduating from college, that I got my chance. I had a job as a counselor at the Hole in the Wall Gang Camp in Ashford, Connecticut. It's a summer camp for children with life-threatening illnesses (primarily cancer and blood disorders). I expected to have a fulfilling summer working with children who needed a break from hospital routines and the chance to be kids. I figured they would also need me to provide support and friendship and, in my case, empathetic understanding. What caught me by surprise was how much I ended up needing them.

Early in the summer I was swimming with several campers in the large pool when Jenny (not her real name), a twelve-year-old girl, noticed something few are able to see, let alone identify. With my hair matted by the water, the "end points" of my craniotomy scar peeked through above my forehead and left ear.

"Hey," she said, with a tone of excitement and surprise, "you had the same surgery I did!"

I didn't hear her clearly amid the splashing and yelling, so I flashed her an automatic smile meant to encourage her delight and enthusiasm over something I assumed was water-related. Jenny, taking her cue from my distant smile, parted her shining brown hair, revealing a beautiful crescent-moon-shaped scar, a reflection of mine.

In three and a half feet of chlorinated water, on a hot July afternoon, surrounded by people of all ages playing, screaming, splashing, Jenny and I embarked on a journey of mutual discovery and exchange. We began by naming our cancers and the degrees of malignancy (usually 1, 2, or 3), and proceeded with animated war stories: the complications, pains, fears, tears, needles, good doctors, scary doctors, unreliable percentages, nausea, hair loss, and radiation.

I wanted to hear from Jenny how she felt about having had cancer, what she had gained and lost from the experience in the years since her ordeal. But I was hesitant. I didn't want, uninvited, to disrupt her fun—after all, we weren't sitting in a circle in a cancer support group. We were swimming in a pool at a camp designed to provide these remarkable children the time of their lives. I settled on the safe route: "Well, how do you feel now, I mean healthwise?"

"Oh, pretty good. I haven't been sick really since the cancer."

"Wonderful," I said. "I've been healthy overall, too, but I'll tell you, Jenny, I'm still trying to make sense of how cancer has changed my life."

She gave me a look that told me she understood. "Yeah, things have never been the same since I got sick—I don't mean really bad—sometimes even good—but definitely different. My whole family thought I was going to die, and then a year later I was healthy and back in school. You should have seen my mom and dad—they were more worried than I was."

"What was it like going back to school after cancer?" I asked.

"Not too bad. At first it was hard. None of my friends knew what it was like. They only knew that I almost died. I hated the hospital, but at least there were people there who understood—you know what I mean?"

I understood all too well. Like Jenny, I was back at school to start my senior year within six months after my radiation treatment ended—from the hospital bed to the dorm room, from death's door to Party Central U.S.A. I was in over my head in a sea of transition and confusion. My return to school, similar to Jenny's, was marked by a deep sense of isolation; very few of my peers could truly understand where I stood, and even fewer wanted to. I didn't blame them. It wasn't long ago that I was one of those cool breeze college kids who had every reason to take living for granted.

To make things worse, my relationship with Rebecca, of nearly three years, was on the rocks, and many of my closest friends had graduated the year before with my original class. I spent much of that first month behind closed doors, reading, working, trying to convince myself that I could manage by using avoidance tactics.

"Well, could you talk to your friends about it?" I asked Jenny.

"Yeah," she replied. "Not at first, though. For a while I just wanted to forget the whole thing. But then I started talking more about it—how scary it was to have surgeries and wait to hear the news from my parents and the doctors, good or bad—you know. I guess that helped. But a few of my friends didn't want to hear it, or maybe they weren't interested. That was weird. It didn't stop me from talking about it; I just went to people who would listen, like my mom and dad, my teacher, and some friends."

Again, this captivating twelve-year-old was describing postcancer life in terms that I could understand. Like Jenny, I had some friends who "didn't want to hear it," avoiding the subject altogether. Maybe they thought that's what I wanted, maybe they were twenty years old and scared; whatever the reason, it marked the beginning of a solitary period of internal and external reevaluation

Because I contemplated death when I did, after twenty-one years of easy living, endangered at most by the occasional breakout of poison oak, my slant on life was shaken. But the challenge came not so much in preparing for death—after all, you have little choice in the matter—as in surviving the ordeal and having to forge a new life. Cancer's presence in my life raised the dust, so to speak, bringing to the surface deeply buried elements of my character. The lenses through which I had always viewed life were changing dramatically. It was up to me to get them into a new focus.

Most apparent and demanding was my need to reconstruct how I thought about relationships. The central theme of my postsurgery psychotherapy was not cancer but cancer's effects on my social interactions. Aided by these sessions, my experience with cancer provided the necessary tools to clarify what I needed from, and offered to, friends, parents, lovers, and people who were yet to enter my life. Cancer became a catalyst, facilitating the adjustment from patient to full-time college student and beyond.

After nearly a month of hiding, I began to open myself to my college community, meeting new people and rekindling old friendships. For example, Rebecca and I built a new relationship based on our shared experiences and the mutual respect we had always had. I surrounded myself with people I thought were emotionally mature and secure, people who weren't afraid to take responsibility for their actions and feelings, people who could weather the thick and the thin. This was important to me because I needed to feel confident that I could rely on my friends to both give and seek support; cancer made me self-protective, but it also enabled me to define and recognize the qualities I most value in friendship.

It turned out that Jenny and I had a lot in common. Our significant age difference, more than a decade, was quite insignificant. Having never discussed recovery experiences with other cancer survivors, I found it was only a matter of minutes before our conversation gave me a new angle. By discussing our similar reactions to cancer and recovery, she had struck a responsive chord. Unwittingly, Jenny helped me develop a language for the experiences I had been sifting and mulling over for the past year. She accomplished this not so much with her words but with her honest approach to understanding and assimilating cancer's presence in her life.

In what proved to be the most rewarding summer of my life, I was fortunate to have many similar exchanges, mostly with children. Time and time again I had the opportunity to delve into the labyrinth of postcancer life. Swapping stories, coping strategies, and insights, we explored new and old territory, steadily learning more about ourselves, more about the process of recovery. The campers exuded a courage and forthrightness that bolstered their ability to face the unfaceable, comprehend the incomprehensible. Like Jenny, they presented a vision both pure and perceptive, uncluttered by the often distracting, obscuring nature of age. These young survivors, offering wisdom for the taking at every turn, inspired me to reach deep within, to initiate a process of renewal that I continue to struggle with.

A group of girls waded their way toward us in the pool, reminding me that Jenny was here to play.

I sensed the depth of our discourse but didn't yet fully understand its magnitude. As she swam away, I mustered a "Thanks."

Already off with her friends, she turned around, grinning.

"Thanks for what?"

Drew's Diet: Nutritional Resources

Appendix A is divided into three sections. The first section is Drew's healing diet; the second lists selected books on natural-foods diets; and the third lists organizations where these books, foods, supplies, and more information can be obtained.

DREW'S HEALING DIET

The following is an exact copy of the diet individually tailored for Drew by a Kushi Institute trained counselor, Evelyne Harborn. It is based on his condition, his general health, his history, and his age. This diet should not be generalized as an "anticancer" diet for all people. It is a strict healing diet designed for Drew when he was most seriously ill.

THE KUSHI FOUNDATION
Macrobiotic Food Selection and Recipe List

For variety, these aspects of day to day cooking can be changed:

1. The selection of foods within the following categories: grains, soups, vegetables, beans, seaweeds, condiments, pickles, and beverages

2. The methods of cooking: boiling, steaming, sauteing, frying, pressure cooking

3. The ways of cutting vegetables

4. The amount of water used

5. The amount of seasoning and condiments used

6. The kind of seasoning and condiments used

7. The length of cooking time (do not overcook or pressure-cook vegetables)

8. The use of higher and lower flame in cooking food

9. The combination of foods and dishes

10. The seasonal cooking adjustments

PREPARATION

Macrobiotic cooking is unique. Simple ingredients in cooking is the key to producing meals that are nutritious, tasty, and attractive. Furthermore, the cook has the ability to change the quality of the food. Stronger cooking, employing greater pressure, salt, heat, and time, makes the energy of food more concentrated; while less pressure, salt, heat, and time makes the energy lighter. A good cook controls these energies, and thereby the health of those for whom he or she cooks, by varying the cooking styles.

METHODS OF COOKING AND FOOD PREPARATION

Regular Use	*Occasional Use*
Pressure cooking	Stir-frying with water
Boiling	*Avoid for 2 months:*
Steaming	Raw
Waterless	Deep-frying
Soup	Tempura
Pickling	Broiling
Water sauteing	Baking
Pressing	

GRAINS

Regular Use	*Occasional Use*
Short-grain brown rice	Sweet brown rice
Medium-grain brown rice	Mochi (pounded sweet rice)
Pearl barley (Hato mugi)	*Avoid:*
Millet	Cracked wheat (bulgur)
Corn	Steel cut oats
Whole-wheat berries	Rolled oats
Rye	Corn grits
Long-grain brown rice	Corn meal
(for hot climates)	Rye flakes
	Couscous

NO BAKED FOODS!

Occasional-Use Flour Products

Twice a week:
  Whole-wheat noodles
  Udon noodles
  Somen noodles

Only if craved:
  Unyeasted whole-wheat bread
  Unyeasted whole-rye bread
  Fu (puffed wheat gluten)
  Seitan (wheat gluten)

GRAIN RECIPES

Brown Rice

1. Soak 2 cups of washed organically grown brown rice in 3 cups of spring water for 3–5 hours (or overnight).

2. Place in a pressure cooker with a pinch of sea salt *or* 1-inch piece of kombu per cup of rice.

3. Bring up to pressure on a medium-high flame.

4. When pressure is up, place a flame deflector underneath, and lower the flame.

5. Cook for 50 minutes.

6. Turn off flame and let the pressure reduce itself naturally.

7. Remove the rice from the pot and put in wooden bowl.

Combinations of Grains

80% brown rice with 20% barley, or 80% brown rice with 20% millet or wheat berries, or corn, etc.

Combinations of Beans

90% brown rice with 10% aduki beans, or 90% brown rice with 10% black soy beans, or chick peas, etc.

Genuine Brown Rice Cream

After surgery.

1. Dry-roast 1 cup of washed brown rice in a cast-iron or stainless-steel skillet until golden brown.

2. Bring rice to a boil with 10 cups of spring water and a pinch of sea salt.

3. Cover; turn on a low flame using a flame deflector.

4. Cook for about 2 hours until water is ½ of the original level.

5. Place the soft brown rice in a cheesecloth or unbleached muslin cloth, tie, and squeeze out the creamy liquid.

6. Reheat the creamy liquid and serve with or without condiment.

7. The rice can also be pressure-cooked for 1 hour with 5 times more water than rice.

SOUP RECIPES

Basic Miso Soup

1 or 2 cups daily.

1. Soak wakame (1½-inch piece per person) for 5 minutes, then cut into small pieces.

2. Add to cold water and bring to a boil. Meanwhile, cut vegetables into small pieces.

3. Add the vegetables to the boiling broth, and boil all together for 2–4 minutes, until vegetables are soft and edible.

4. Dilute miso (½ to 1 flat teaspoon per cup of broth), add to soup, and *simmer* for 3–4 minutes on a low flame.

5. Occasionally, a small portion of shiitake mushrooms can be cooked in with the other vegetables.

Note: Please vary the type of vegetables every day, and include leafy greens often.

Thick Miso Soup with Daikon and Mochi

Often.

Use the same recipe as above, allowing the daikon to get soft. Add leafy green vegetables toward the end of cooking. Occasionally, sliced tofu or mochi can be added before adding the miso.

Other Soup Suggestions

A) Grain Vegetable Soup:
   Add leftover cooked grains to basic miso soup, or make fresh millet or barley soup with vegetables.

B) Bean Vegetable Soup:
   Add leftover cooked beans to basic miso soup, or make a fresh soup using lentils or precooked beans.

C) Squash Soup:
   Cut and cook squash in water until it dissolves. Season with a pinch of sea salt or a dash of tamari.

Soup Seasoning Suggestions

A) *Light* use of tamari soy sauce

B) *Light* use of salt

Note: Add small amounts of fresh garnish when serving soup (e.g., chopped parsley or scallions). Please try to have fresh soup every day and avoid using too many leftovers.

Ojiya: Rice and Miso Stew. Once a day for a few days after surgery.

VEGETABLES

REGULAR USE	OCCASIONAL USE	AVOID:
Green Leafy	Celery	Artichoke
Carrot tops	Chives	Avocado
Collard Greens	Cucumber	Bamboo shoots
Dandelion leaves	Endive	Beets
Kale	Escarole	Curley dock
Leeks	Green beans	Eggplant
Mustard greens	Green peas	Fennel
Parsley	Iceberg lettuce	Ferns
Watercress	Jerusalem artichoke	Ginseng
Bok Choy	Kohlrabi	Green/Red pepper
Chinese cabbage	Mushrooms	New Zealand spinach
	Patty pan squash	Okra
Round	Romaine lettuce	Plantain
Acorn squash	Salsify	Purslane
Broccoli	Snap beans	Shepherd's purse
Brussels sprouts	Snow peas	Potato
Butternut squash	Sprouts	Sorrel
Buttercup squash	Summer squash	Spinach
Shiitake mushrooms	Wax beans	Sweet potato
Cabbage		Swiss chard
Cauliflower		Tomato
Hubbard squash		Taro potato—albi
Hokkaido pumpkin		Yams
Onion		Zucchini
Pumpkin		
Red cabbage		
Rutabaga		
Turnip		

Appendix A

Root

Burdock
Carrots
Daikon
Dandelion roots
Jinenjo
Lotus root
Parsnips
Radish

VEGETABLE RECIPES

3 to 4 dishes a week

Nishime Dish (Waterless Cooking)

1. Use a heavy pot with a heavy lid or cookware specifically designed for waterless cooking.

2. Soak a 3-inch piece of kombu until soft and cut into 1-inch-square pieces.

3. Place kombu in bottom of pot and cover with water (about 1–2 inches of water).

4. Add sliced vegetables. For nishime preparation, vegetables are cut in large sizes. It is usually a combination of 2 or 3 vegetables, such as carrots, daikon, turnip, burdock root. It may also include onions, hard winter squash, or cabbage.

5. The vegetables can be layered in the pot, on top of the kombu, or placed in sections around the pot.

6. Sprinkle a few pinches of sea salt or tamari over the vegetables.

7. Cover and set the flame on high until a good steam is generated. Lower the flame and simmer for 15–20 minutes. If the water should evaporate too quickly during cooking, add more water to the bottom of the pot.

8. When each vegetable has become soft and edible, add a few drops of tamari and toss the pot (do not stir).

9. Cover and cook over a low flame for 3–5 minutes.

10. Remove lid, turn off flame, and let the vegetables sit for about 2 minutes. You may serve the vegetable juice along with the dish.

Nishime Combination Suggestions

A) Carrot, burdock, and kombu

B) Burdock, lotus root, and kombu

C) Daikon, lotus root, and kombu

D) Carrot, parsnip, and kombu

E) Turnip, shiitake mushrooms, and kombu

F) Squash, onion, and kombu

Note: There are several other combinations. It is not advisable to cook only carrot and daikon or carrot and turnip unless one is using other vegetables as well.

Squash (60%), Aduki Beans (30%), and Kombu (10%) Dish
2 or 3 times a week

1. Wash and soak ½ cup of aduki beans with 1-inch-square piece of kombu for 2–5 hours.

2. Place kombu in the bottom of the pot, and add chopped hard winter squash such as acorn, butternut, or buttercup (or hokkaido). When squash is not available, substitute onions, carrots, or parsnips.

3. Add aduki beans on top of squash and cover with water.

4. Cook over a low flame until the beans and squash become soft. You may need to add cold water a few times during cooking.

5. When the beans are 80% done, add a few pinches of sea salt.

6. Cover and cook for another 10–15 minutes or until all the water has cooked down.

7. Turn off the flame, and let the pot sit for several minutes before serving.

Note: During cooking it is best not to stir the beans at all.

Dried Daikon with Kombu with Onions and Carrots
1 cup 2 times a week; can be in Nishime.

1. Soak a 2-inch piece of kombu for 10 minutes. Slice it into ½-inch pieces and place in the bottom of a pot that has a heavy lid.

2. Soak ½ cup of dried daikon for about 10 minutes or until it is soft. If the dried daikon is a very dark color, discard the soaking water.

3. Place dried daikon on top of the kombu.

4. Add kombu soaking water and enough additional water to just cover the daikon.

5. Cover the pot, bring to a boil, and lower the flame. Simmer for about 30–40 minutes, until the daikon is tender.

6. Add a small amount of tamari, and cook away the excess liquid.

Note: You may sometimes add other vegetables, such as onion or carrots, at the beginning of the cooking.

Appendix A

Daikon and Daikon Leaves, or Carrots and Carrot Tops, or Turnip and Turnip Greens, or Dandelion Roots and Dandelion Leaves

Often.

1. Finely chop one of the suggestions above.

2. Place in a pot with a small volume of water.

3. Cover and cook with steam for about 10 minutes.

4. Toward the end of cooking, add a small pinch of sea salt or a small amount of tamari, and simmer for 2–4 minutes.

Note: You may lightly cook the root part first and add the leafy part later.

Boiled Salad (Blanched Vegetables)

Almost daily.

When making boiled salad, boil each vegetable separately, one at a time but in the same water. Cook the mildest-tasting vegetables first so that each vegetable will retain its distinctive flavor. Any combination of 2–3 vegetables may be used, but make sure it varies each time. For this short, 1-minute-cooking style, the vegetables must be chopped finely (matchsticks or thin slices).

1. Place several inches of water and a pinch of sea salt in a pot and bring to a boil.

2. Drop in a small amount of vegetables at a time and allow to boil for 1 minute. Remove the vegetables quickly from the water and place them in a strainer.

3. Repeat step 2 with each kind of vegetable. When done, transfer them into a serving dish.

Note: The vegetables in this dish are fresh and crispy. They may be served plain or with a few drops of vinegar (brown rice or umeboshi) or with several pinches of condiment.

Pressed Salad (Quick Pickling)

Twice a week if desired.

1. Wash and slice desired vegetables into very thin pieces (i.e., red radishes, cabbage, celery, cucumbers, carrots, daikon, or vegetable leaves).

2. Place vegetables in a pickle press or large bowl and sprinkle about ½ teaspoon of sea salt per cup of chopped vegetables. Mix gently by hand.

3. Apply pressure to the press. If you are using a bowl, place a small plate on top of the vegetables and a weight on top of the plate.

4. Let it sit for 1 hour or more (depending on the vegetables) or until the water has come out of the vegetables.

5. Before serving, discard the water and carefully wash off the salt.

Raw Salad

None for now.
A variety of vegetables may be used in this preparation: cabbage, grated carrots, radishes, cucumbers, celery, watercress, etc.

Salad Dressing Suggestions

A) 1 umeboshi plum or 1 teaspoon of umeboshi paste, added to $\frac{1}{2}$ teaspoon of miso and puréed in a suribachi.

B) Dilute miso in warm water and heat for a few minutes. Add a few drops of rice vinegar.

C) Gomashio or shiso leaf powder.

D) Sprinkle a few drop of umeboshi vinegar.

E) Add a few drops of tamari and lemon juice.

Steamed Green Dish

Almost daily.

1. Wash and slice any of the following vegetables: turnip greens, daikon greens, carrot tops, kale, mustard greens, watercress, collard greens, chinese cabbage, etc.

2. Place vegetables in a small amount of boiling water ($\frac{1}{2}$ inch) or in a stainless-steel steamer over 1 inch of boiling water.

3. Cover and steam for 2–3 minutes, depending on the texture of the vegetables.

4. At the end of the cooking, lightly sprinkle tamari over the vegetables.

5. Transfer quickly into a serving dish.

Note: When served, greens should still be fresh and bright.

Sauteed Vegetables (with Water)

2–3 times a week.

1. Cut carrots, onions, cabbage (finely cut), or other vegetables, including leafy greens.

2. Brush the bottom of the pan with dark sesame oil, or put in a small amount of water. When hot, sauté the vegetables quickly for a few minutes. Sprinkle with a pinch of salt or tamari, and add a little water if necessary.

3. Simmer for a few more minutes. The vegetables should be crispy and colorful, but cooked.

Kinpira

⅔ cup, 2–3 a week.

1. Lightly brush sesame oil in a skillet and heat up.

2. Place equal amounts of burdock and carrots (cut up into matchsticks or shaved) into the skillet, and add a pinch of sea salt.

3. Sauté for 2–3 minutes.

4. Lightly cover the bottom of the skillet with water. Cover and cook until the vegetables are 80% done; this should be about 30 minutes or more.

5. Add several drops of tamari, cover, and cook until all the water has cooked down.

6. At the very end of cooking, *add a few drops of ginger juice (from grated ginger)*.

Note: Onions, turnips, or dried lotus root can be substituted or used together with carrots and burdock.

Dried Tofu, or Tofu, or Tempeh, or Seitan (after one month), with Vegetables (Stew Type)

2 or 3 times a week.

1. Soak a 2-inch piece of kombu in 3 cups of water.

2. Bring to a boil and cook for 3–5 minutes.

3. Add either one of the following: soaked and sliced dried tofu or tempeh cubes or cooked seitan, along with sliced daikon, burdock, carrots, or lotus root to the boiling water and cook for about 15 minutes.

4. If you use cooked seitan, you may not need to add any additional salt or tamari. If you use tempeh or dried tofu, you may want to add a pinch of sea salt of a dash of tamari.

5. Add a combination (2 or 3) of the following vegetables: onions, cabbage or chinese cabbage, squash, or brussels sprouts, and cook for 3–5 minutes.

6. If you use fresh tofu, add in the lighter green vegetables toward the end of the cooking.

7. Chop finely 2 or 3 scallions and cook in for about 1 minute.

Note: All the vegetables should be boiled or cooked until soft, but the leafy greens should still be crisp. A small amount of ginger may be added at the very end of cooking. A mild seasoning of miso may be added at the end of cooking, instead of tamari.

BEANS

Regular Use (day-to-day OK)

Aduki beans
Chick peas (garbanzo beans)
Lentils (green-brown)
Black soybeans

Bean Products

Dried tofu
Fresh tofu
Tempeh

Occasional Use (2–3 times a month)

Black-eyed peas
Black turtle beans
Great Northern beans
Kidney beans
Lima beans
Mung beans
Navy beans
Pinto beans
Soybeans
Split peas
Whole dried peas

BEAN RECIPES

Beans can be cooked in the following ways:

A) with kombu (10%)

B) with carrots and onions (20%)

C) with acorn/butternut or buttercup squash (30–50%)

D) with chestnuts (10–30%)

E) in soup with other vegetables

F) with grains (10%)

SEA VEGETABLES

Sea vegetables are used frequently in soups, vegetable dishes, and bean dishes, or they are cooked as a side dish.

Regular Use

Toasted nori sheet
Wakame (daily)
Kombu (daily)

Optional Use

Agar-agar (gelatin)
Dulse
Irish moss
Mekabu
Sea palm

Occasional use (twice a week)

Arame
Hiziki

155

Appendix A

CONDIMENTS

Main Condiments (moderate)

Gomashio (sesame seeds with sea salt)
Seaweed powder with or without toasted sesame seeds
Shiso leaves powder ($\frac{1}{4}$ teaspoon a day)
Tekka
Umeboshi plums
Green nori flakes

Other Condiments

Brown rice vinegar
Cooked miso with scallions
Nori condiment
Shio kombu
Umeboshi plum with scallions
Umeboshi vinegar
Shiso leaves powder with toasted sesame seeds

CONDIMENT RECIPES

Umeboshi Plum

Small piece ($\frac{1}{4}$ plum) daily.

Umeboshi plums can be purchased in natural foods stores.

Gomashio (Toasted Sesame Seeds with Sea Salt)

1 tsp. a day.

The standard ratio for gomashio is 1 part salt to 18 parts sesame seeds; however, this can be altered according to various needs. Black sesame seeds are preferred to yellow ones.

1. In a stainless-steel skillet, toast the sea salt for a few minutes until it is shiny. Then grind the salt down in a suribachi until it is very fine.

2. Place washed sesame seeds in the skillet and toast on a low-medium flame, stirring constantly with a wooden spoon, shaking the skillet from time to time. When the seeds give off a nutty fragrance and begin popping, crush one between the thumb and the small finger. If it crushes easily, they are done.

3. Place the seeds in the suribachi containing the ground sea salt. Slowly grind the seeds, using an even circular motion until the seeds are half crushed.

4. Allow to cool and store in a covered glass jar.

Kombu or Wakame Seaweed Powder and (Optional) Toasted Sesame Seed
¼ tsp. a day

1. Roast seaweed in a dry skillet until it is dark and crisp.

2. Grind into a fine powder in a suribachi.

Note: If you are adding the sesame seeds, toast them according to the directions in the gomashio recipe. Then add them to the seaweed powder and crush them together. The ratio of seaweed to sesame seeds can be ⅔ seaweed to ⅓ sesame seeds.

Tekka
This condiment is made from 1 cup of minced burdock, lotus root, carrots, miso, sesame oil, and ginger flavor. It can be made at home, or bought ready-made.

PICKLES

Regular Use

Bran pickles (Nuka)
Brine pickles (water/salt)
Miso bean pickles
Miso pickles
Pressed pickles
Sauerkraut
Tamari pickles
Takuan pickles (with daikon)

Note: A small amount of daikon pickles, natural sauerkraut, and other natural pickles can be used, almost daily, in a small volume. However, if they are too salty, you may rinse them or soak them in water for 10 minutes.

PICKLE RECIPES

Umeboshi Pickles

1. Place 6–8 umeboshi plums in a large jar. Add 2 quarts of water.

2. Shake and let sit for a few hours, until the water turns pink.

3. Place sliced vegetables in the water. Cover with a cheesecloth, and place the jar in a dark, cool place.

4. Serve after 4–5 days.

Quick Tamari Pickles

1. Slice root or round vegetables ⅛ inch thick and cover with a mixture of 50% water and 50% tamari.

2. After 2 hours (or less, if onions), remove vegetables from the liquid and serve. If the taste is too salty, rinse the vegetables off.

3. Save the liquid for future pickling.

Tamari Pickles

1. Mix water ⅔ water and ⅓ tamari in a bowl or glass jar.

2. Add sliced root and round vegetables.

3. Keep in a cool and dark place and serve after 5 days or more.

Brine Pickles

1. Boil 3 cups of water and 1 teaspoon of sea salt. Let cool.

2. Place a 3-inch piece of kombu and slices of carrots, onion, daikon, broccoli, cauliflower, cucumber, etc. in a jar with the cool salt water. All the vegetables should be immersed in the salt water; if not, place a smaller jar or cup inside to press the vegetables below the surface of the water.

3. Cover with a cheesecloth and keep in a cool place for 2–3 days.

4. Refrigerate and start using when the vegetables have lost their raw flavor but still retain their crunchiness.

OCCASIONAL FOODS

WHITE MEAT FISH

When needed; may be once a week.

Carp	Trout
Cod	Red Snapper
Haddock	Sole
Halibut	Flounder
Scrod	

and any other *soft* white meat fish.

FISH SOUP RECIPE

Koi-Koku: Carp with Burdock or Trout with Carrots

If necessary for vitality.

1. Buy a fresh carp, preferably not frozen.

2. Ask the fish seller to carefully remove the gallbladder and yellow bitter bone (thyroid) and leave the rest of the fish intact. This includes all scales, bones, head, and fins.

3. At home, chop the entire fish into 2–3-inch slices. Remove the eyes if you wish.

4. Meanwhile, chop at least an equal amount of burdock (equal to the weight of the fish) into thinly shaved slices or matchsticks. This quantity of burdock may take a while to prepare.

5. When everything is chopped, place the burdock and fish in a pressure cooker.

6. Tie bancha twigs (about 1 cup) in a cheesecloth. Place it in the pressure cooker on top or nestled inside the fish. The tea twigs will help soften the bones while cooking.

7. Add enough liquid to cover the fish and burdock, approximately ⅓ bancha tea and ⅔ spring water. Pressure cook for 1 hour to 1½ hour.

8. Bring the pressure down, take off the lid and replace on a low flame. Add miso to taste (as you would for regular miso soup) and a small amount of grated ginger juice.

9. Simmer for 5 minutes. Garnish with chopped scallions and serve hot. If fresh carp is not available, trout may be substituted. In this case, carrots can be used instead of burdock.

FRUIT

Only if craved; otherwise, none.
Cooked, dried, or, if permitted, fresh seasonal northern-climate fruit.

Tree Fruit	*Ground Fruit*
Apples	Blueberries
Apricots	Blackberries
Cherries	Cantaloupe
Grapes	Honeydew melon
Peaches	Raspberries
Pears	Strawberries
Plums	Watermelon
Tangerines	
Raisins or currants	

Note: Use a pinch of sea salt in cooked fruits and on raw fruits. Avoid all tropical fruits.

NUTS

Occasional Lightly Roasted Nontropical Nuts	*Avoid All Tropical Nuts*
Chestnuts	Brazil nuts
	Cashews
	Hazel nuts
	Macadamia nuts
	Pistachio nuts

Appendix A

SEEDS

Occasional Lightly *Roasted, Unsalted Seeds*:
Up to 1 cup a week.

Pumpkin seeds
Sesame seeds

SNACKS

Mochi	Seeds
Rice balls	Popcorn
Noodles	Rice cakes
Leftovers	Puffed whole cereal grains
Sushi (homemade)	

SWEETS

A sweet taste can be achieved with the following vegetables:
Cabbage
Carrots
Daikon
Onions
Parsnips
Squash
Chestnuts
Sweet vegetable drink (see recipe)
Sweet vegetable jam

Other possible sweets:

Once a week:
Amasake

Moderate:
Barley malt
Brown rice syrup

Only very occasionally:
Hot apple juice
Hot apple cider

SEASONINGS

Regular Use	*Occasional Use*	*Avoid*:
Barley miso (Mugi miso)	Ginger	All commercial
Soybean miso (Hatcho miso)	Horseradish	seasonings and all
Tamari soya sauce (shoyu)	Rice vinegar	spices or herbs.
Unrefined *white* sea salt	Umeboshi vinegar	
	Umeboshi plum	
	Umeboshi paste	
	Garlic (cooked)	
	Lemon (only for fish)	

BEVERAGES

Regular Use	*Occasional Use*
Bancha stem tea	Grain coffee (100% grain)
Bancha twig tea (Kukicha)	Dandelion tea
Roasted barley tea	Kombu tea
Roasted brown rice tea	Umeboshi tea
Spring water	Mu tea
Well water	Carrot juice
Sweet vegetable drink	Celery juice
(1 cup a day)	

Infrequent Use	*Avoid*:
Green tea	Distilled water
Barley sprouts powder	Coffee
Vegetable juice	Cold drinks (with ice cubes)
Northern climate fruit juice	Hard liquors
Beer	Herb teas
Sake (hot or cold)	Mineral water and all bubbling water
Whiskey	(Carbonated)
Soy milk (with kombu)	Regular tea
	Stimulant beverages
	Aromatic beverages
	Sugared and soft drinks
	Tap water
	Wine

Appendix A

Sweet Vegetable Drink

1 cup a day.

1. Chop finely: ¼ cup of onions, ¼ cup of carrots, ¼ cup of cabbage, and ¼ cup of squash (sweet winter squash).

2. Add to boiling water (4 cups) and allow to boil for 2–3 minutes. Reduce flame to low, cover, and let simmer for 20 minutes.

3. Strain out vegetables (you may use them in soups or stews).

4. Drink the broth hot or warm or at room temperature.

Note: No seasoning is used in this recipe. Sweet vegetable broth may be kept in the refrigerator, but warm it up again before drinking or let it come back to room temperature.

HOME REMEDIES

The following home preparations are safe, simple, and effective traditional remedies that have been used by people throughout the Orient for many generations.

INTERNAL PREPARATIONS

Tamari-bancha tea

Ume-sho-bancha

Ume-sho-kuzu

Ume-sho-kuzu and ginger

Sweet vegetable drink

Carrot-daikon drink

Mu tea

Umeboshi tea

Umeboshi-bean tea

Azuki-bean tea

Fresh lotus root tea

Shiitake Mushroom tea

Kombu tea

Tamari-Bancha Tea

To strengthen the blood if an overly acidic condition exists, to relieve fatigue, to relieve headaches due to an overly yin or overly acidic condition, to stimulate good blood circulation.

1. Place 1 teaspoon of tamari in a teacup and pour in hot bancha tea.

2. Stir and drink while hot.

Ume-Sho-Bancha

1 cup a day for 3 days.
To strengthen the blood, regulate digestion and circulation, to relieve fatigue and weakness, to relieve various types of sicknesses caused by overconsumption of yin foods or beverages.

1. Place ½ umeboshi plum in a teacup with ½ teaspoon of tamari.

2. *Pour in hot bancha tea and stir well. Drink hot.*

Ume-Sho-Kuzu

Once a week for 3 weeks (after surgery).
To strengthen digestion and restore energy, to strengthen intestinal condition; good for stomach problems.

1. Dilute 1 heaping teaspoon of kuzu with a couple of teaspoons of water.

2. Add diluted kuzu to 1 cup of water.

3. Add the meat of ½–1 umeboshi plum to the water and kuzu.

4. While bringing to a boil, stir constantly to avoid lumping. Reduce flame and simmer until it is translucent.

5. Add ½–1 teaspoon of tamari and stir. Simmer ½ minute longer. Drink it while it is hot.

Ume-sho-Kuzu with Ginger

Same use as plain Ume-sho-kuzu, but more yin in preparation. Prepare in the same manner as above, but add ⅛ teaspoon of fresh grated ginger at the same time the tamari is added.

Mu Tea

For digestive problems (e.g., a weak stomach), for respiratory problems (e.g., coughing), for reproductive disorders (e.g., menstrual cramps or irregular menstruation).
Mu tea is composed of a combination of 16 plants and wild herbs. The drink is a combination of yin and yang ingredients, but as a whole it is a yang drink.
A less yang Mu tea drink, containing only 9 of those plants and more or less similar to the original herbal drink, is available.

Umeboshi Tea

This is a very refreshing drink for the summer.

1. Boil the meat of 1 umeboshi for ½ hour in 1 quart of water.

2. Strain and, if necessary, dilute with more water.

3. Let cool and drink.

Appendix A

Carrot-Daikon (or Lotus) Drink

1 cup every 3 days for 1 month.
This drink helps to dissolve solidified fat deposits existing deep within the body.

1. Grate ½ cup of carrots, plus ½ cup of daikon.
2. Add 2 cups of water and simmer 4 minutes. Add a few drops of soy sauce *or* a pinch of sea salt while simmering.

Aduki Bean Tea

Treats kidney problems, constipation.

1. Place 1 cup of beans in a pot and add 3–4 times more water and one 7–8-inch strip of kombu.
2. Bring to a boil.
3. Reduce flame to low; cover and simmer for 45 minutes to 1 hour.
4. Strain out the beans and drink the liquid hot.

Shiitake Mushroom Tea

To reduce fevers in small children and babies, to help discharge animal foods, to help discharge toxins in boils caused by the overconsumption of animal foods, to help generally relax from a contracted condition.

1. Place 1 cup of water and 1 shiitake mushroom in a saucepan.
2. Bring to a boil.
3. Reduce flame and simmer several minutes.
4. Add a drop of tamari and drink while hot.

Fresh Lotus Root Tea

Once a week for 1 month.
To *relieve mucus in lungs, to relieve coughing and sinuses.*

1. Wash lotus root.
2. Grate ½ cup of lotus root. Place pulp in a piece of cheesecloth and squeeze out the lotus juice.
3. Place the juice in a saucepan.
4. Add enough water to equal the same amount of lotus juice.
5. Add a pinch of sea salt, bring to a boil, reduce the flame and let it simmer for a few minutes.

Note: This drink should be very thick and creamy.

Sweet Vegetable Drink

This drink is good for people suffering from hypoglycemia, tight pancreas, stomach and spleen problems.

1. Use equal amounts of 4 sweet vegetables (e.g., carrot, squash, onion, and cabbage).

2. Add four times more water than vegetables.

3. Bring to a boil and then simmer for 10–15 minutes.

4. Strain; drink 1–2 cups a day.

Kombu Tea

Strengthens the blood, helps clean out animal fats and proteins, helps restore the nervous system.

1. Boil a 3-inch strip of kombu in a quart of water until only half the water is left (about 10 minutes).

2. Drink 2–3 cups per day.

EXTERNAL TREATMENTS

Body scrub daily, morning and evening

SELECTED BOOKS ON NATURAL-FOODS DIETS

I have divided the following books into two categories. First are books that explain the principles of natural foods and health, particularly macrobiotics—the why's of healthy eating. These books are primarily food theory but include some recipes. The second category is cookbooks—the how-to's of eating well and deliciously. Although these books concentrate on cooking, they also include some of the rationales for healing diets.

Selected Books about Healthy Eating

Colbin, Annemarie. *Food and Healing.* Ballantine Books, 1986.
Kushi, Michio. *The Macrobiotic Way: The Complete Diet and Exercise Book.* Avery, 1985.
Kushi, Michio, with Alex Jack. *Cancer Prevention Diet.* St. Martin's Press, revised and updated, 1993.
Robbins, J. *Diet for a New America.* Stillpoint Publishing, 1987.
Rogers, Sherry A. *The Cure Is in the Kitchen.* Prestige Publishing, 1990 (1-800-846-6687).
———. *You Are What You Ate.* Prestige Publishing, 1988 (1-800-846-6687).

Appendix A

Selected Cookbooks

Colbin, Annemarie. *The Book of Whole Meals.* Ballantine Books, 1979.
————. *The Natural Gourmet.* Ballantine Books, 1991.
Estella, Mary. *Natural Foods Cookbook: Vegetarian Dairy-Free Cuisine.* Japan Publications, 1985.
Gallinger, Shirley, and Sherry A. Rogers. *Macro Mellow.* Prestige Publishing, 1992 (1-800-846-6687).
Kushi, Aveline, and Wendy Esko. *The Quick and Natural Macrobiotic Cookbook.* Contemporary Books, 1989.
Kushi, Aveline, with Alex Jack. *Complete Guide to Macrobiotic Cooking for Health, Harmony and Peace.* Warner Books, 1985.
Turner, Kristina. *The Self-Healing Cookbook.* Earthtones Press, 1987.
Vegetarian Journal's Guide to Natural Foods Restaurants in the U.S. and Canada, 1-800-548-5757 (in case you get tired of cooking).

MAIL ORDER COMPANIES

The following are a few relevant phone numbers and addresses for ordering the above books, foods, and supplies.

The Kushi Foundation Store
P.O. Box 7
Becket, MA 01223
(413) 623-2102
You can order the numerous Kushi-authored books from this number as well as an array of health-related texts and supplies. The Kushi Institute also publishes a newsletter reviewing new books, offering recipes, and highlighting new medical research on food and health: *One Peaceful World Newsletter,* (413) 623-2322.

Mountain Ark Trading Company
Fayetteville, AR 72701
1-800-643-8909
(foods, equipment, and books)

Natural Lifestyle Supplies
Asheville, NC 28804
1-800-752-2775
(foods, equipment, and books)

Diamond Organics
Box 2159
Freedom, CA 95019
1-800-922-2396
(organic produce shipped fresh)

Walnut Acres
Penns Creek, PA 17862
1-800-433-3998
(organic foods, many prepared)

Aveline's Natural Food Store
42 Park Street
Lee, MA 01238
(413) 243-1775
(foods, equipment, and books)

Gold Mine Natural Foods of San Diego
1947 30th Street
San Diego, CA 92102
1-800-475-3663
(foods, equipment, and books)

EDUCATIONAL RESOURCES AND REFERRALS

Following are references for further information on nutritional counseling
and education.

The Kushi Institute (Michio and Aveline Kushi)
P.O. Box 7
Becket, MA 01223
(413) 623-5742
The Kushi Institute offers educational programs at the Becket headquarters.
Staff members will discuss your concerns over the phone and refer you to
nutritional counselors in your area.

Commonweal (Michael Lerner)
P.O. Box 316
Bolinas, CA 94924
(415) 868-0970

The Natural Gourmet Cooking School (Annemarie Colbin)
48 West 21st Street, Second Floor
New York, NY 10010
(212) 645-5170
You can take classes here, for an afternoon or several weeks, on healthy
cooking in general or for a specific illness. Annemarie Colbin is available for
health consultations.

Appendix A

George Ohsawa Macrobiotic Foundation (Herman and Cornellia Aihara)
1511 Robinson Street
Oroville, CA 95965
(916) 533-7702
The Aiharas offer macrobiotic counseling, referrals, and educational healing programs.

Sherry A. Rogers, M.D.
Northeast Center for Environmental Medicine
2800 West Genesee Street
Syracuse, NY 13219
Sherry Rogers publishes a newsletter on environmental health updates: Prestige Publishing, Box 3638, Syracuse, NY 13220; 1-800-846-6687.

National Environmental Health Association
720 South Colorado Blvd., Suite 970
Denver, CO 80222
(303) 756-9090
This organization publishes the *Journal of Environmental Health*, provides education and credentials for environmental health–related specialists, holds conferences, and is a clearinghouse for publications on the subject.

The Human Ecology Action League
P.O. Box 49126
Atlanta, GA 30359-1126
(404) 248-1898
This national organization publishes *The Human Ecologist*, a quarterly magazine on environmental health.

The Human Ecology Action League of Central New York
3773 Dorothy Drive
Syracuse, NY 13215
(315) 492-0091
HEAL of CNY publishes a newsletter on environmental health that focuses on environmental illness but includes environment-related health concerns such as cancer. The phone contact people are helpful, informative, and supportive.

APPENDIX B
Mind/Body Connections

SELECTED READINGS

Books

Benson, Herbert. *Beyond the Relaxation Response*. Random House, 1984.
Borysenko, Joan. *Minding the Body, Mending the Mind*. Bantam Books, 1988.
Goleman, Daniel, and Joel Gurin. *Mind/Body Medicine: How to Use Your Mind for Better Health*. Consumer Reports Books, 1993.
Kabat-Zinn, Jon. *Full Catastrophe Living*. Delacorte Press, 1990. Audiotapes available: Stress Reduction Tapes, P.O. Box 547, Lexington, MA, 02173.
_____. *Wherever You Go, There You Are: Mindfulness Meditation in Everyday Life*. Hyperion, 1994.
Locke, Steven, and Douglas Colligan. *The Healer Within*. Dutton, 1986.
Moyers, Bill. *Healing and the Mind*. Doubleday, 1993.
Rossman, Martin L. *Healing Yourself: A Step-by-Step Program for Better Health through Imagery*. Walker, 1987. Audiotapes available: Insight Publishing, P.O. Box 2070, Mill Valley, CA 94942; (415) 388-8225.
Spiegel, David. *Living beyond Limits: New Hope and Help for Facing Life Threatening Illness*. Times Books, 1993.
Thich Nhat Hanh. *The Miracle of Mindfulness: A Manual on Meditation* (rev. ed.). Beacon Press, 1993.

Newletters

Circle of Healing, edited by Joan Borysenko and Miron Borysenko, Mind/Body Health Sciences, Inc.; (303) 440-8460.
Mental Medicine Update: The Mind/Body Health Newsletter, edited by David Sobel; 1-800-222-4745.

Appendix B

STRESS REDUCTION CENTERS

The following are a few among many such centers proliferating around the country. To find one in your area, consult your local hospital or call one of the centers below for a referral.

Stress Reduction Clinic (Jon Kabat-Zinn, Ph.D.)
University of Massachusetts Medical Center
Worcester, MA 01655
(508) 856-1616
(videotapes available)

David Spiegel, M.D.
Stanford University School of Medicine
Psychiatry and Behavioral Sciences
Stanford, CA 94305
(415) 723-6421

Preventive Medicine Research Institute (Dean Ornish, M.D.)
University of California, School of Medicine
900 Bridgeway, Suite 2
Sausalito, CA 94965
(415) 332-2525

The following four centers are affiliated with each other:

Mind/Body Medical Institute (Herbert Benson, M.D.)
New England Deaconess Hospital
Department of Behavioral Medicine
110 Francis Street, Suite 1A
Boston, MA 02215
(617) 632-9525

Behavioral Medicine
Mercy Hospital and Medical Center
Stevenson Expressway at King Drive
Chicago, IL 60662
(312) 567-2259

Mind/Body Medical Institute
Morristown Memorial Hospital
95 Mt. Kemble Avenue
Morristown, N.J. 07962
(201) 971-4575

Mind/Body Medical Institute
Memorial Health Care Systems
7500 Beechnut Street, Suite 321
Houston, TX 77074
(713) 776-5020

APPENDIX C

Chinese and Holistic Medicine

SELECTED BOOKS

(Listed are general reference guides to books on acupuncture and Chinese medicine, herbal medicines, and Ayurvedic methods)

Beinfeld, Harriet, and Efrem Korngold. *Between Heaven and Earth: A Guide to Chinese Medicine* Ballantine Books, 1991.

Bensky, D., and A. Gamble. *Chinese Herbal Medicine—Materia Medica* (rev. ed.). Eastland Press, 1993; Box 12689, Seattle, WA 98111.

Cargill, Marie. *Acupuncture: A Viable Medical Alternative: A Layperson's Guide* Greenwood, 1994.

Chopra, Deepak. *Ageless Body, Timeless Mind: The Quantum Alternative to Growing Old.* Crown, 1993.

Dharmananda, S. *A Bag of Pearls.* Institute for Traditional Medicine and Preventive Health Care, 1992; 2017 Southeast Hawthorne, Portland, OR 97214; 1-800-544-7504. (A newsletter on using herbs and acupuncture to treat diseases such as AIDS and cancer can also be ordered from this institute.)

Firebrace, Peter. *Acupuncture: The Illustrated Guide.* Harmony Books, 1988.

Kaptchuk, Ted. *The Web That Has No Weaver: Understanding Chinese Medicine.* Congdon and Weed, 1984.

Kaptchuk, Ted, and Michael Croucher. *The Healing Arts: Exploring the Medical Ways of the World.* Summit, 1987.

Kastner, Mark, and Hugh Burroughs. *Alternative Healing: The Complete A–Z Guide to Over 160 Different Alternative Therapies.* Halcyon, 1993.

Lerner, Michael. *Choices In Healing: Integrating the Best of Conventional and Alternative Approaches to Cancer.* MIT Press, 1994.

Lowenberg, June S. *Caring and Responsibility: The Crossroads Between Holistic Practice and Traditional Medicine.* University of Pennsylvania Press, 1989.

McIntyre, Anne. *Herbal Medicine.* Tuttle Alternative Health Series, 1993.

Monte, Tom. *World Medicine: The East-West Guide to Healing Your Body.* Tarcher/Putnam, 1993.

Moss, Ralph W. *Cancer Therapy: The Independent Consumer's Guide to Non-Toxic Treatment and Prevention.* Equinox, 1993.

Naeser, Margaret. *Outline Guide to Chinese Herbal Patent Medicines in Pill Form—with Sample Pictures of the Boxes: An Introduction to Chinese Herbal Medicines.* Boston Chinese Medicine, 1990; Box 5747, Boston, MA 02114.

Tierra, Michael. *Planetary Herbology: An Integration of Western Herbs into the Traditional Chinese and Ayurvedic Systems.* Lotus Press, 1988.

Walters, Richard. *Options: The Alternative Cancer Therapy Book.* Avery, 1993.

Williams, David, M.D., *Alternatives: For the Health Conscious Individual,* Mountain Home Publishing, P.O. Box 829, Ingram, TX 78025; 1-800-527-3044.

Holistic Health Directory (published by *New Age Journal*; 1-800-782-7006) lists types of care and practitioners by state and is issued annually.

ORGANIZATIONS

American Association of Acupuncture and Oriental Medicine
433 Front Street
Catasauqua, PA 18032-2506
(610) 433-2448
AAAOM offers nationwide referrals to state and local associations as well as individual practitioners. They work on insurance coverage and lobby in Washington for Oriental medicines.

American Holistic Medical Association
4101 Lake Boone Trail, Suite 201
Raleigh, NC 27607-6518
(919) 787-5181
AHMA offers the same services as AAAOM.

NOTES

Chapter 2. I've Never Heard That One Before (pages 14–28)

1. Yvonne Daly, *The Boston Sunday Globe*, August 23, 1992.
2. *Boston Globe*, November 16, 1993.
3. *Boston Globe*, August 6, 1992. Rita Arditti with Tatiana Schreiber, "Breast Cancer: The Environmental Connection," *Resist* (newsletter), May/June 1992, pp. 1–9.
4. Nancy Sokol Green, *Poisoning Our Children: Surviving in a Toxic World* (Chicago: Noble Press, 1991).
5. R. H. Fletcher and S. W. Fletcher, "Clinical Research in General Medical Journals: A 30-year Perspective," *New England Journal of Medicine* 301 (1979): 180–83.
6. Alex Jack, lecture, Kushi Institute, June 1991.

Chapter 3. And Please, No More One Percent Odds (pages 29–52)

1. J. Teas, M. L. Harbison, and R. S. Gelman, "Dietary Seaweed and Mammary Carcinogenesis in Rats," *Cancer Research* 44 (1984): 2758–61.
2. Steven A. Rosenberg, "Combined Modality Therapy for Cancer," *New England Journal of Medicine* 312 (1985): 1512–14; Alex Jack, ed., *Let Food Be Thy Medicine* (Becket, Mass.: One Peaceful World Press, 1991).

3. Herman Melville, *White Jacket: Or the World in a Man of War* (New York: New American Library, 1981), p. 253.

Chapter 4. Surgery Two (pages 53–69)

1. Bobbie Ann Mason, *Spence and Lila* (New York: Harper and Row, 1988), p. 20.
2. John Dundas, *The Boston Workout* (Needham, Mass.: Chestnut Hill Press [P. O. Box 826, Needham, Mass. 02192], 1993).
3. H. Bursztajn, R. I. Feinbloom, R. M. Hamm, and A. Brodsky, *Medical Choices, Medical Chances: How Patients, Families, and Physicians Can Cope with Uncertainty* (New York: Routledge, 1990).
4. Vincent T. DeVita, Jr., M.D., et al., *Cancer: Principles and Practice of Oncology*, 3rd ed., vol. 1 (Philadelphia: J. B. Lippincott Company, 1989); National Cancer Institute, *Bone Cancers* (research report, NIH Publication No. 91–721) (Bethesda, Md.: NCI, 1990).
5. K. H. Antman, et al., "Soft Tissue Sarcoma: Current Trends in Diagnosis and Management," *Current Problems in Cancer* 13 (1989): 33–67.
6. Kenneth R. Pelletier, Ph.D., quoted in Martin L. Rossman, Ph.D., *Healing Yourself: A Step-by-Step Program for Better Health Through Imagery* (New York: Walker and Co., 1987).
7. Sarah Arsone, with Carolyn Reuben, "Nonsurgical Care for Fibroids," *Ms.*, December 1988, p. 27.

Chapter 5. Americans Can't Eat This Way (pages 70–86)

1. H. D. Suit, et al., "Increased Efficacy of Radiation Therapy by Use of Proton Beam," *Strahlentherapie Onkologie* 166 (1) (1990): 40–44.
2. M. Austin Seymour, et al., "Considerations in Fractionated Proton Radiation Therapy: Clinical Potential and Results," *Radiotherapy and Oncology* 17 (1990): 29–35.
3. John Robbins, *Diet for a New America* (Walpole, N.H.: Stillpoint Publishing, 1987).
4. Ibid; Annemarie Colbin, *Food and Healing* (New York: Ballantine Books, 1986).
5. *Boston Globe*, September 10, 1993.
6. *Healthy People: The Surgeon General's Report on Health Promotion and Disease Prevention* (Washington, D.C.: Government Printing Office, 1979).
7. United States Senate Select Committee on Nutrition and Human Needs, *Dietary Goals for the United States*, 95th Cong., 1st sess., 1977 (rev. 1980).
8. Edward Esko, ed., *Doctors Look at Macrobiotics* (New York: Japan Publications, 1988), p. 12.
9. National Academy of Sciences, *Diet, Nutrition and Cancer* (Washington D.C.: National Academy Press, 1982).

10. Robert McCarrison, M.D., "Faulty Food in Relation to Gastro-Intestinal Disorder," *Journal of the American Medical Association* 78 (1922): 1–8.

11. W. E. Connor, et al., "The Plasma Lipids, Lipoproteins, and Diet of the Tarahumara Indians of Mexico," *American Journal of Clinical Nutrition* 31 (1978): 1131–42.

12. D. M. Ingram, "Trends in Diet and Breast Cancer Mortality in England and Wales, 1928–1977," *Nutrition and Cancer* 3 (1981): 75–80.

13. F. M. Sacks, et al., "Effects of Ingestion of Meat on Plasma Cholesterol of Vegetarians," *Journal of the American Medical Association* 246 (1981): 640–44.

14. Patricia Anstett, *Boston Globe*, April 19, 1992.

15. Dean Ornish, M.D., *Dr. Dean Ornish's Program for Reversing Heart Disease* (New York: Random House, 1990).

16. Elaine Nussbaum, *Recovery from Cancer to Health through Macrobiotics* (New York, Japan Publications, 1985), p. 82; reprint, Garden City, N.Y.: Avery Publishing Group, 1993).

17. Tatsuichiro Akizuki, "How We Survived Nagasaki," *East West Journal*, December 1980, quoted in Alex Jack (ed.), *Let Foods Be Thy Medicine* (Becket, Mass.: One Peaceful World Press, 1991), pp. 87–88.

18. "Miso Protects against Radiation," *Yomiuri Shinbun*, July 16, 1990.

19. "Miso Shows Promise as Treatment for Radiation," *Japan Times*, September 27, 1988.

20. S. C. Skoryna, et al., "Studies on Inhibition of Intestinal Absorption of Radioactive Strontium: 1. Prevention of Absorption from Ligated Intestinal Segments," *Canadian Medical Association Journal* 91 (1964): 285–88.

21. Y. Tanaka, et al., "Studies on Inhibition of Intestinal Absorption of Radioactive Strontium: 7. Relationship of Biological Activity to Chemical Composition of Alginates Obtained from North American Seaweeds," *Canadian Medical Association Journal* 99 (1968): 169–75.

22. Y. Tanaka, et al., "Studies on Inhibition of Intestinal Absorption of Radioactive Strontium: 9. Relationship between Biological Activity and Electron Microscope Appearance of Alginic Acid Components," *Canadian Medical Association Journal* 103 (1970): 484–486.

23. Christiane Northrop, M.D., "Cancer Revisited—Seven Years Later," in Edward Esko, ed., *Doctors Look at Macrobiotics* (New York: Japan Publications, 1988), pp. 67, 69–70.

24. Jean Craig, *Between Hello and Goodbye: A Life-Affirming Story of Courage in the Face of Tragedy* (Los Angeles: Jeremy P. Tarcher, 1991).

Chapter 6. Western Reflections on Eastern Medicine (pages 87–115)

1. Edie Magnus, "CBS Evening News," October 21, 1992.

2. Ibid., October 25, 1992.

3. Bill Moyers, *Healing and the Mind* (New York: Doubleday, 1993).

4. For example, Anastacia Toufexis, "Dr. Jacobs' Alternative Mission," *Time*, March 1, 1993, pp. 43–44. "Can Your Mind Heal Your Body?" *Consum-*

er Reports, January 1994, pp. 51–59. Arielle Emmet, "Where East Does Not Meet West," *Technology Review*, November/December 1992, pp. 50–56.

5. David M. Eisenberg, M.D., et al., "Unconventional Medicine in the United States: Prevalence, Costs, and Patterns of Use," *New England Journal of Medicine* 328 (1993): 246–52.

6. Ralph W. Moss, *The Cancer Industry: Unravelling the Politics* (New York: Paragon Press, 1989), p. xxi.

7. Kit Kitatani, "Stomach Cancer," in Ann Fawcett and Cynthia Smith, eds., *Cancer Free: 30 Who Triumphed over Cancer Naturally* (New York: Japan Publications, 1991), p. 107.

8. Anthony J. Sattilaro, M.D., *Recalled by Life* (New York, Avon Books, 1982).

9. Michael Shanik, "Malignant Melanoma," in Ann Fawcett and Cynthia Smith, eds., *Cancer Free* (New York: Japan Publications, 1991), pp. 47, 51.

10. Dirk Benedict, *Confessions of a Kamikaze Cowboy* (Garden City, NY: Avery Publishing Group, 1991), p. 64.

11. Sattilaro, *Recalled by Life*, p. 182.

12. Hugh Faulkner, M.D., "Pancreatic Cancer," in Ann Fawcett and Cynthia Smith, eds., *Cancer Free* (New York: Japan Publications, 1991), p. 144.

13. Dr. Hugh Faulkner, *Physician Heal Thyself* (Becket, Mass.: One Peaceful World Press, 1992).

14. Faulkner, "Pancreatic Cancer," in Ann Fawcett and Cynthia Smith, eds., *Cancer Free* (New York: Japan Publications, 1991), p. 148.

15. American Cancer Society, *Cancer Facts and Figures*, 1992. National Cancer Institute, interview by author with Angela Harris, February 7, 1994.

16. Steven A. Rosenberg, "Combined-Modality Therapy of Cancer," *New England Journal of Medicine* 312 (1985): 1512–14.

17. John Cairns, "The Treatment of Diseases and the War Against Cancer," *Scientific American*, November 1985, pp. 51–59. See also Moss, *The Cancer Industry*.

18. Richard Knox, *Boston Globe*, January 26, 1994.

19. John C. Bailar III and Elaine M. Smith, "Progress against Cancer," *New England Journal of Medicine* 314 (1986): 1226–32.

20. Victor Herbert, M.D., J.D., "Unproven (Questionable) Dietary and Nutritional Methods in Cancer Prevention and Treatment," *Cancer* 58 (1986): 1930–41.

21. Barrie R. Cassileth, Ph.D., et al., "Survival and Quality of Life among Patients Receiving Unproven as Compared with Conventional Cancer Therapy," *New England Journal of Medicine* 324 (1991): 1180–85.

22. For example, Johanna T. Dwyer, "Unproven Nutritional Remedies and Cancer," *Nutritional Reviews* 50 (April 1992): 106–109.

23. Barrie R. Cassileth, Ph.D., and Deborah Berlyne, Ph.D., "Counseling the Cancer Patient Who Wants to Try Unorthodox or Questionable Therapies," *Oncology* 3 (April 1989): 29–33.

24. Editors, "Unproven Methods of Cancer Management— Macrobiotic Diets," *CA* 34 (January/February 1984): 60–63.

25. Cathy Arnold, "The Macrobiotic Diet: A Question of Nutrition," *Oncology Nursing Forum* 11 (May/June 1984): 50–53.

26. U.S. House, Subcommittee on Health and Long-Term Care, "Quackery: A $10 Billion Scandal" (Washington, D.C.: U.S. Government Printing Office, 1984): pp. 66–68, 107. (Committee Publication No. 94–435).

27. Michael Lerner, Ph.D., "The Article Reviewed," *Oncology* 3 (April 1989): 34, 40–41.

28. *Boston Globe*, May 20, 1992.

29. Paolo Toniolo, et al., "Calorie-Providing Nutrients and Risk of Breast Cancer," *Journal of the National Cancer Institute* 81 (1989): 278–86; Walter Troll, "Prevention of Cancer by Agents That Suppress Oxygen Radical Formation," *Free Radical Research Communications* 12–13 (1991): 751–57; Walter C. Willet, M.D., et al., "Dietary Fat and Fiber in Relation to Risk of Breast Cancer," *Journal of the American Medical Association* 268 (1992): 2037–44 (see also accompanying editorial, pp. 2080–81).

30. L. A. Cohen, et al., "Modulation of N-nitrosomethylurea-induced Mammary Tumor Promotion by Dietary Fiber and Fat," *Journal of the National Cancer Institute* 83 (1991): 496–501.

31. J. E. Baggott, et al., "Effect of Miso (Japanese Soybean Paste) and NaCl on DMBA-induced Rat Mammary Tumors," *Nutrition and Cancer* 14 (1990): 103–9.

32. Ichiro Yamamoto, et al., "The Effects of Dietary Seaweeds on 7,12-dimethyl-benz[a]anthracene-induced Mammary Tumorigenesis in Rats," *Cancer Letters* 35 (1987): 109–18; J. Teas, M. L. Harbison, and R. S. Gelman, "Dietary Seaweed and Mammary Carcinogenesis in Rats," *Cancer Research* 44 (1984): 2758–61.

33. J. Raloff, "A Soy Sauce Surprise," *Science News* 139 (1991): 357.

34. T. Hirayama, "Epidemiology of Stomach Cancer," in T. Murakami ed., *Early Gastric Cancer*, Gann Monographs on Cancer Research, no. 11 (Tokyo: University of Tokyo Press, 1971), pp. 3–19.

35. Vivien Newbold, M.D., "Remission of Cancer Patients on a Macrobiotic Diet," unpublished paper.

36. Office of Technology Assessment (OTA), "Unconventional Cancer Treatments" (Washington, D.C.: Government Printing Office, 1990).

37. James P. Carter, et al., "Hypothesis: Dietary Management May Improve Survival from Nutritionally Linked Cancers Based on Analysis of Representative Cases," *Journal of the American College of Nutrition* 12 (1993): 209–26.

38. Barrie R. Cassileth, et al., "Psychosocial Correlates of Cancer Survival: A Subsequent Report 3 to 8 Years after Cancer Diagnosis," *Journal of Clinical Oncology* 6 (1988): 1753–59; Laurence T. Vollhardt, "Psychoneuroimmunology: A Literature Review," *American Orthopsychiatric Association* 61 (1991): 35–47.

39. Jon Kabat-Zinn, Ph.D., *Full Catastrophe Living: Using the Wisdom of Your Body and Mind to Face Stress, Pain and Illness* (New York: Dell, 1990), pp. 181–82.

40. Steven E. Locke, M.D., and Douglas Colligan, *The Healer Within: The New Medicine of Mind and Body* (New York: E. P. Dutton, 1986).
41. Janice K. Kiecolt-Glaser, et al., "Modulation of Cellular Immunity in Medical Students," *Journal of Behavioral Medicine* 9 (1986): 5–21.
42. Ibid.; Janice Kiecolt-Glaser and Ronald Glaser, "Major Life Changes, Chronic Stress, and Immunity," in T. Peter Bridge, et al., eds., *Psychological, Neuropsychiatric, and Substance Abuse Aspects of AIDS* (New York: Raven Press, 1988); Janice Kiecolt-Glaser and Ronald Glaser, "Psychoneuroimmunology: Past, Present, and Future," *Health Psychology* 8 (1989): 677–82.
43. Kabat-Zinn, *Full Catastrophe Living*, J. Bernhard, et al., "Effectiveness of Relaxation and Visualization Techniques as an Adjunct to Phototherapy and Photochemotherapy of Psoriasis," *Journal of the American Academy of Dermatology* 19 (1988): 572–73.
44. Kabat-Zinn, *Full Catastrophe Living*, p. 209.
45. Ibid.
46. *One Peaceful World*, no. 10, Spring 1992, "Medical-Scientific Update," p. 3.
47. Margaret A. Naeser, Ph.D., Dip. Ac., et al., "Real versus Sham Acupuncture in the Treatment of Paralysis in Acute Stroke Patients: A CT Scan Lesion Site Study," *Journal of Neurologic Rehabilitation* (forthcoming).
48. Kabat-Zinn, *Full Catastrophe Living*, p. 192.
49. Milton L. Bullock et al., "Controlled Trial of Acupuncture for Severe Recidivist Alcoholism," *Lancet*, June 24, 1989, pp. 1435–39.
50. Christopher Boyd, *Boston Globe*, April 17, 1992.
51. *One Peaceful World*, no. 10, Spring 1992, "Medical-Scientific Update," p. 3.
52. Nancy Waring, *The Boston Globe Magazine*, June 17, 1990.
53. Ibid.
54. *Boston Globe*, August 7, 1992.

Chapter 7. Robust Resistance (pages 116–137)

1. Ann Fawcett and Cynthia Smith, *Cancer-Free: 30 Who Triumphed Over Cancer Naturally* (New York: Japan Publications, 1991), p. 110.
2. Ibid., p. 189.
3. Elaine Nussbaum, *Recovery from Cancer to Health through Macrobiotics* (New York: Japan Publications, 1986, p. 205; reprint, Garden City, N.Y.: Avery Publishing, 1993).
4. John Steel Gordon, "How America's Health Care Fell Ill," *American Heritage* 43 (May/June 1992): 49–65.
5. Oliver Wendell Holmes, "The Contagiousness of Puerperal Fever," *New England Quarterly Journal for Medicine and Surgery* (1843), in *Medical Classics*. 1 (November 1936): 213.
6. Alexandra Dundas Todd, *Intimate Adversaries: Cultural Conflict between Doctors and Women Patients* (Philadelphia: University of Pennsylvania

Press, 1989), and "Ending the War on Disease," *Socialist Review* 20 (July–September 1990): 99–114.

7. Sir W. J. Sinclair, *Semmelweiss: His Life and His Doctrine* (Manchester: The University Press, 1909).

8. Thomas S. Kuhn, *The Structure of Scientific Revolutions* (Chicago: University of Chicago Press, 1962).

9. Joseph Lister, "On the Antiseptic Principle of the Practice of Surgery," *British Medical Journal* (1867), in *Medical Classics* 2 (September 1937): 83.

10. Perri Klass, *A Not Entirely Benign Procedure: Four Years as a Medical Student* (New York: Signet, 1987).

11. Judy Foreman, *Boston Globe*, February 1, 1989. See also Vincent Castronova, Claude Colin, Bernadette Parent, Jean-Michel Foidart, Rene Lambotte, and Phillippe Mahiew, "Possible Role of Human Natural Anti-Gal Antibodies in the Natural Antitumor Defense System," *Journal of the National Cancer Institute* 81 (1989): 212–16.

12. Jeanette Winterson, *Written on the Body* (New York: Alfred A. Knopf, 1993).

13. Rita Arditti with Tatiana Schreider, "Breast Cancer: The Environmental Connection," in *Resist* (newsletter), no. 246, May/June 1992, pp. 1–9.

14. Alan Bennett, *The Madness of George III*, performed at the Colonial Theater, Boston, November 12, 1993. From *The Madness of George III* by Alan Bennett (London: Faber and Faber, 1992), p. 51.

15. Elizabeth Kubler-Ross quoted in Christiane Northrup, M.D., "Cancer Revisited—Seven Years Later," in Edward Esko, ed., *Doctors Look at Macrobiotics*, (New York: Japan Publications, 1988), p. 71.

16. Vivien Newbold, M.D., F.A.C.E.P., "Macrobiotics: An Approach to the Achievement of Health, Happiness and Harmony," in Edward Esko, ed., *Doctors Look at Macrobiotics*, (New York: Japan Publications, 1988), p. 47.

17. Anthony J. Sattilaro, M.D., *Recalled by Life* (New York: Avon Books, 1982), pp 178–79.

18. Ibid., p. 178.

19. Judith Glassman, quoted in Northrup, "Cancer Revisited," in Edward Esko, ed., *Doctors Look at Macrobiotics* (New York: Japan Publications, 1988), p. 67.

20. E. Mumford, H. J. Schlesinger, and G. V. Glass, "The Effect of Psychological Intervention on Recovery from Surgery and Heart Attacks: An Analysis of the Literature," *American Journal of Public Health* 72 (1982): 141–51.

21. D. Breen, *The Birth of a First Child: Towards an Understanding of Femininity* (London: Tavistock, 1975); J. M. Levy and R. K. McGee, "Childbirth as Crises: A Test of Janis' Theory of Communication and Stress Resolution," *Journal of Personality and Social Psychology* 29 (1974): 710–18.

22. J. E. Johnson and H. Leventhal, "Effects of Accurate Expectations and Behavioral Instructions of Reactions during a Noxious Medical Examination," *Journal of Personality and Social Psychology* 29 (1974): 710–18.

23. J. A. Wolfer and M. A. Vistainer, "Pediatric Surgical Patients of Psychologic Preparation and Stress-Point Nursing Care," *Nursing Research* 24 (1975): 244–55.

24. Stephen Jay Gould, *The Mismeasure of Man* (New York: Norton, 1981), p. 21.

25. Guillermo Asis, M.D., "Awakening to Common Sense," in Edward Esko, ed., *Doctors Look at Macrobiotics*, (New York: Japan Publications, 1988), p. 172.

26. Marc Van Cauwenberghe, M.D., "A Macrobiotic Way of Healing," in Edward Esko, ed., *Doctors Look at Macrobiotics* (New York: Japan Publications, 1988), p. 115.

27. Henry Edward Altenberg, M.D., "My Explorations in Macrobiotics," in Edward Esko, ed., *Doctors Look at Macrobiotics* (New York: Japan Publications, 1988), p. 135.

28. Helen V. Farrell, M.D., "PMS Is Not PMS," in Edward Esko, ed., *Doctors Look at Macrobiotics* (New York: Japan Publications, 1988), pp. 177–91.

29. Terry Shintani, M.D., J.D., M.P.H., "Macrobiotics, Nutrition, and Disease Prevention," in Edward Esko, ed., *Doctors Look at Macrobiotics* (New York: Japan Publications, 1988), pp. 193–206.

30. Anatole Broyard, *Intoxicated by My Illness* (New York: Clarkson Potter/Publishers, 1992), p. 47.

31. Ibid., p. 45.

32. Rita Charon, M.D., "Doctor-Patient/Reader-Writer: Learning to Find the Text," *Soundings* 72 (Spring 1989): 1101–16.

33. David Dodson, M.D., "Diet—the Best Medicine," in Edward Esko, ed., *Doctors Look at Macrobiotics* (New York: Japan Publications, 1988), p. 141.

34. Shintani, "Macrobiotics," in Edward Esko, ed., *Doctors Look at Macrobiotics* (New York: Japan Publications, 1988), p. 193.

Conclusion (pages 138–140)

1. Tim O'Brien, *The Things They Carried* (New York: Penguin Books, 1990), pp. 219–20.

INDEX

Index

RECIPE INDEX

The following foods usually can be obtained in health food stores, and through the mail order companies listed in Appendix A.

UNIVERSITY PRESS OF NEW ENGLAND
publishes books under its own imprint and is the publisher for
Brandeis University Press, Brown University Press, University of
Connecticut, Dartmouth College, Middlebury College Press,
University of New Hampshire, University of Rhode Island,
Tufts University, University of Vermont, Wesleyan University
Press, and Salzburg Seminar.

ALEXANDRA TODD is Professor of Sociology at Suffolk
University. She is the author of numerous articles on the social
aspects of health care and most recently of the book *Intimate
Adversaries: Cultural Conflict between Doctors and Women Pa-
tients*. She has edited, with Sue Fisher, *Gender and Discourse:
The Power of Talk* and *The Structure of Discourse and Institution-
al Authority: Law, Medicine, Education*. She currently lives in
Boston, Massachusetts.

LIBRARY OF CONGRESS CATALOGING-IN-PUBLICATION DATA
Todd, Alexandra Dundas.
  Double vision : an East-West collaboration for coping with cancer
/ Alexandra Dundas Todd.
      p.   cm.
  Includes index.
  ISBN 0-8195-5279-8
  1. Todd, John Andrew—Health. 2. Brain—Cancer—Patients—
United States—Biography. 3. Cancer—Alternative treatment.
I. Title.
  [DNLM: 1. Todd, John Andrew. 2. Neoplasms—therapy—popular
works. 3. Patients—biography. 4. Medicine, Oriental Traditional.
QZ 201 T633d 1994]
RC280.B7T63 1994
362.1'96994'0092—dc20
[B]
DNLM/DLC
for Library of Congress   94-8013
♾